LIFESTYLE
OBESITY MANAGEMENT

LIFESTYLE OBESITY MANAGEMENT

Edited by

John P. Foreyt, PhD
Professor
Department of Medicine
Director, Behavioral Medicine Research Center
Baylor College of Medicine
Houston, Texas

Kyle J. McInnis, ScD
Associate Professor
Department of Exercise Science and Physical Education
University of Massachusetts
Boston, Massachusetts

Walker S. Carlos Poston II, PhD, MPH
Mid America Heart Institute and
University of Missouri-Kansas City
Kansas City, Missouri

James M. Rippe, MD
Founder and Director
Rippe Lifestyle Institute
Shrewsbury, MA
Associate Professor of Medicine
Tufts University School of Medicine
Boston, Massachusetts
Founder and Director
Rippe Health Assessment at Celebration Health
Orlando, Florida

Part of the *Lifestyle Medicine Series*, edited by James M. Rippe

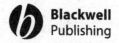

Blackwell
Publishing

© 2003 by James M. Rippe

Blackwell Publishing, Inc., 350 Main Street, Malden, Massachusetts 02148-5018, USA
Blackwell Publishing Ltd, 9600 Garsington Road, Oxford OX4 2DQ, UK
Blackwell Publishing Asia Pty Ltd, 550 Swanston Street, Carlton South, Victoria 3053, Australia
Blackwell Verlag GmbH, Kurfürstendamm 57, 10707 Berlin, Germany

02 03 04 05 5 4 3 2 1

ISBN: 1-4051-0344-2

Library of Congress Cataloging-in-Publication Data
Lifestyle obesity management / John P. Foreyt . . . [et al.].
        p. ; cm.
    Includes bibliographical references and index.
    ISBN 1-40510-344-2 (pbk.)
    1. Obesity.   2. Health behavior.
3. Lifestyles.
    [DNLM: 1. Obesity—etiology.
2. Obesity—therapy. WD 210 L722 2003]   I. Foreyt, John Paul.
RC628 .L474 2003
616.3'98—dc21   2002012475

A catalogue record for this title is available from the British Library
Acquisitions: Jim Krosschell
Development: Amy Nuttbrock
Production: Lorna Hind
Manufacturing: Lisa Flanagan
Marketing: Jeanne Fryar
Cover design: Calvin Nelson

For further information on Blackwell Publishing, visit our website:
http://www.blackwellpublishing.com

Contents

List of Contributors   vii

Preface   xii

1.   Modern Management of Obesity:
The Value of a Multidisciplinary Approach   1
**Kathleen J. Melanson, Kyle J. McInnis,
and James M. Rippe**

2.   Exercise Management of the Obese
Patient   34
**David Neubauer Lombard and
Tamara Neubauer Lombard**

3.   Dietary Management of the
Obese Patient   58
**Sachiko St. Jeor, Judith M. Ashley,
and Jon P. Schrage**

4. Behavioral Strategies for Enhancing Weight Loss and Maintenance   85
Teresa K. King, Elizabeth E. Lloyd-Richardson, and Matthew M. Clark

5. Drug Treatment of Obesity   106
William W. Hardy and Nikhil V. Dhurandhar

6. Surgery for Morbid Obesity   138
Harvey J. Sugerman, Eric J. DeMaria, and John M. Kellum

7. Managing Obesity to Lower the Risk of Cardiovascular Disease and Other Chronic Conditions   156
Kathleen J. Melanson, James B. Meigs, Kyle J. McInnis, and James M. Rippe

8. Childhood Obesity   193
Scott Owens and Bernard Gutin

9. Obesity and Health: Public Policy Implications and Recommendations   224
Kathleen J. Melanson, Kyle J. McInnis, and James M. Rippe

10. Obesity Research in the New Millennium   251
Risa J. Stein, C. Keith Haddock, Walker S. Carlos Poston II, and John P. Foreyt

Index   269

List of Contributors

Judith M. Ashley, PhD, RD
Nutrition Education and Research Program
Department of Internal Medicine
University of Nevada School of Medicine
Reno, Nevada

Matthew M. Clark, PhD
Department of Psychology
The Mayo Clinic
Rochester, Minnesota

Eric J. DeMaria, MD
Medical College of Virginia
Virginia Commonwealth University
Richmond, Virginia

Nikhil V. Dhurandhar, PhD
Department of Nutrition and Food Science
Wayne State University
Detroit, Michigan

John P. Foreyt, PhD
Professor
Department of Medicine
Director, Behavioral Medicine Research Center
Baylor College of Medicine
Houston, Texas

Bernard Gutin, PhD
Professor
Georgia Prevention Institute
Medical College of Georgia
Augusta, Georgia

C. Keith Haddock, PhD
Department of Psychology
University of Missouri-Kansas City
Kansas City, Missouri

William W. Hardy, MD
Rochester Center for Obesity Research
Rochester Hills, Minnesota

John M. Kellum, MD
Medical College of Virginia
Virginia Commonwealth University
Richmond, Virginia

Teresa K. King, PhD
Brown University Center for Behavioral and
    Preventative Medicine
The Miriam Hospital
Providence, Rhode Island

Elizabeth E. Lloyd-Richardson, PhD
Brown University Center for Behavioral and
  Preventative Medicine
The Miriam Hospital
Providence, Rhode Island

David Neubauer Lombard, PhD
Parkview Behavioral Health
Parkview Health System
Fort Wayne, Indiana

Tamara Neubauer Lombard, PhD
Parkview Behavioral Health
Parkview Health System
Fort Wayne, Indiana

Kyle J. McInnis, ScD
Associate Professor
Department of Exercise Science and
  Physical Education
University of Massachusetts
Boston, Massachusetts

James B. Meigs, MD, MPH
General Internal Medicine
Massachusetts General Hospital
Boston, Massachusetts

Kathleen J. Melanson, PhD, RD
Department of Nutrition and Food Sciences
University of Rhode Island
Kingston, Rhode Island

Scott Owens, PhD
Department of Health and Human Performance
Western Carolina University
Cullowhee, North Carolina

Walker S. Carlos Poston II, PhD, MPH
Mid America Heart Institute and
    University of Missouri-Kansas City
Kansas City, Missouri

James M. Rippe, MD
Founder and Director
Rippe Lifestyle Institute
Shrewsbury, Massachusetts and Associate
    Professor of Medicine
Tufts University School of Medicine
Boston, Massachusetts and
Founder and Director
Rippe Health Assessment at Celebration
Health
Orlando, Florida

Jon P. Schrage, MD
Nutrition Education and Research Program
Department of Internal Medicine
University of Nevada School of Medicine
Reno, Nevada

Sachiko St. Jeor, PhD, RD
Nutrition Education and Research Program
Department of Internal Medicine
University of Nevada School of Medicine
Reno, Nevada

Risa J. Stein, PhD
Department of Psychology
Rockhurst College
Kansas City, Missouri

Harvey J. Sugerman, MD
Medical College of Virginia
Virginia Commonwealth University
Richmond, Virginia

Preface

By any criteria, overweight and obesity represent major health challenges to the United States and to the rest of the industrialized world. Twenty-six percent of the adult population in the United States is currently obese and 35% of the adult population is at least somewhat overweight. Moreover, the prevalence of obesity grew an astounding 40% in the last decade for which there are good data available. Perhaps even more alarmingly, the prevalence of childhood and adolescent obesity has more than doubled over the past 20 years.

Obesity contributes in significant ways to coronary heart disease, diabetes, various gastrointestinal diseases, osteoarthritis, and many other chronic conditions. Obesity (along with its twin epidemic of physical inactivity) in the United States represents the second leading cause of preventable mortality each year behind only cigarette smoking. Underlying causes of obesity include genetic propensity, inadequate physical activity and poor nutritional habits. A wide variety of complex behaviors contributes to the development of both childhood and adult obesity.

For all of these reasons, the editors felt the time had come to assemble a monograph for physicians and other healthcare professionals summarizing current knowledge about the causes and treatments of obesity with an emphasis on lifestyle practices and habits and their contribution to the prevention and treatment of this condition. What has resulted is our book, *Lifestyle Obesity Management.*

Some of the material in this book was originally published as a section edited by two of us (JF, WCP) of a larger textbook, *Lifestyle Medicine*, edited by another (JMR). Additional material was drawn from other sections of this larger textbook. In addition, new chapters were written emphasizing the value of a multidisciplinary approach to obesity treatment as well as approaches to managing obesity to lower the risk of cardiovascular disease and other chronic conditions. All chapters taken from our previous work have been extensively updated and expanded to include new information in the rapidly growing field of obesity treatment. The positive response to various chapters on obesity from our previous textbook as well as the desire to make this material available to a wider audience who might not be interested in all of the topics included in the larger textbook, prompted us to gather this material in the current monograph. It is our hope and intention that this book will serve as a useful guide to all healthcare professionals representing the diverse disciplines required to effectively treat obesity.

Lifestyle Obesity Management is the second in a series of books related to lifestyle issues and their impact on both short and long-term health and quality of life. Much as in the previous monograph that was published, *Lifestyle Nutrition* edited by Dr. Rippe and Dr. Johanna Dwyer, our intention was to provide state-of-the-art understandings of how various aspects of lifestyle practices and habits interact with health.

We wish to acknowledge the excellent efforts of a variety of individuals who have contributed to *Lifestyle Obesity Management*. First we wish to acknowledge and thank our collaborating authors: Kathleen J. Melanson, Tamara Neubauer Lombard, David Neubauer Lombard, Sachiko St. Jeor, Judith M. Ashley, Jon P. Schrage, Teresa K. King, Elizabeth E. Lloyd-Richardson, Matthew M. Clark,

William W. Hardy, Nikhil V. Dhurandhar, Harvey J. Sugerman, Eric J. DeMaria, John M. Kellum, James B. Meigs, Scott Owens, Bernard Gutin, Risa J. Stein, and C. Keith Haddock, all of whom made superb contributions.

Secondly, no textbook, even one that is relatively small such as this would be possible without the superb editorial efforts and coordination of Dr. Rippe's Editorial Director, Elizabeth Porcaro, who guides all aspects of editorial production at *Rippe Lifestyle Institute*. Carol Moreau, Dr. Rippe's Executive Assistant, keeps a complex lifestyle moving forward while freeing time to allow Dr. Rippe to write and edit a variety of scholarly works.

Our longtime friends and colleagues at Blackwell Publishing have been very supportive of both this book and the entire category of lifestyle medicine. We wish to particularly acknowledge James Krosschell, Senior Vice President and Publisher, without whose support the publication of these books would not have been possible.

Finally, we wish to gratefully acknowledge the multiple contributions of our families whose understanding, love and support continues to allow the generation of scholarly works and make all of our efforts worthwhile. Dr. Rippe's wife, Stephanie Hart Rippe and his four young daughters, Hart Elizabeth Rippe, Jaelin Davis Rippe, Devon Marshall Rippe and Jamie Conrad Rippe provide the loving and supportive environment enabling scholarly and other efforts. Dr. McInnis' wife Susan and their three children Brendan, Riley, and Shane who provide love, support, encouragement, laughter, and joy.

It is our hope that *Lifestyle Obesity Management* will continue to advance the multidisciplinary field of obesity management. It is only through the collaboration of dedicated professionals in diverse fields that we will begin to reverse the alarming epidemic of obesity in the United States and other industrialized countries.

John Foreyt, PhD
Walker Carlos Poston, PhD
Kyle McInnis, ScD
James Rippe, MD

Notice: The indications and dosages of all drugs in this book have been recommended in the medical literature and conform to the practices of the general community. The medications described do not necessarily have specific approval by the Food and Drug Administration for use in the diseases and dosages for which they are recommended. The package insert for each drug should be consulted for use and dosage as approved by the FDA. Because standards for usage change, it is advisable to keep abreast of revised recommendations, particularly those concerning new drugs.

Chapter 1

Modern Management of Obesity: The Value of a Multidisciplinary Approach

Kathleen J. Melanson, Kyle J. McInnis, and James M. Rippe

This new century brings growing challenges and opportunities for health professionals who assist individuals in body weight management, as well as for scientists seeking to advance knowledge regarding obesity, energy balance regulation and optimal health. Of serious concern from a clinical and public health standpoint is the escalation of the obesity epidemic (1–4), and its effects on multiple chronic diseases (5,6) (see also Chapter 7), economic burdens (7), and quality of life (8,9).

Scientific and clinical evidence is accumulating to support the importance and efficacy of multidisciplinary strategies in body weight management (2,10). Because obesity is multifactorial in nature, a multidisciplinary approach is most appropriate, and has the highest likelihood of success (11). Such an approach encompasses every aspect of body weight and health, including nutrition, physical activity, behavior, and other factors that may influence these. An integrated team of health care professionals consisting of physicians, nurses, dietitians, exercise physiologists, and behaviorists provides the optimal approach to healthful weight management (12). Of particular importance in this approach is the focal point of health outcomes, individualized treatment addressing the specific needs of each person separately and the emphasis on permanent changes in overall lifestyle rather than a quick fix or magic bullet (2). This chapter provides a systematic formulation of potential multidisciplinary strategies to treating obese patients, discussing the roles of each member of the multidisciplinary team, and interactions among team members. It starts with discussions of the definition of obesity, followed by an overview of the current status and changing trends in obesity and weight management. The position of obesity as a medical condition, and multidisciplinary approaches to obesity treatment and lifestyle weight management will then be described in detail.

DEFINING AND ASSESSING OBESITY

Rather than expressing body mass as "percentage ideal weight", body mass index (BMI) has become the accepted method both clinically and scientifically as a preferable indicator of relative adiposity (1,2). BMI is defined as weight in kilograms divided by height in meters squared: $BMI = kg/m^2$. BMI can be calculated in Imperial units by multiplying weight in pounds by 704.5, and dividing by height in inches squared. BMI conversions in metric and Imperial units are shown in Table 1-1A and 1-1B.

BMI provides a single number that can be broadly applied and is inexpensive enough for clinical use, as well as for large population studies. In dealing with individuals, it must be kept in mind that BMI criteria are based on population data. Limitations of BMI include that it does not distinguish fat mass from lean mass. BMI may not accurately reflect total body fat in all individuals, such as very muscular people (highly trained athletes) and those with very high bone density (e.g. males of African descent), or individuals with edema or postural abnormalities. Clinical judgment must be used in interpreting BMI in such circumstances (2). Additionally, BMI does not provide an estimate of body fat distribution, which is of significance in determining risk for metabolic diseases (13) (see also Chapter 7). Despite some limitations, BMI remains a convenient and useful estimate of adiposity and has been widely accepted in population-based studies to estimate health risks by relative body weight and body fat for some. Clinically, BMI provides a practical determinant of weight-related health risk, which can be employed as a basis for recommendations and assessments.

The World Health Organization (WHO) and National Institutes of Health (NIH) have established criteria of overweight to be defined as BMI levels of 25.0–29.9 kg/m^2 and obesity as BMI ≥ 30.0 kg/m^2 (Table 1-2). Obesity is further subcategorized as Class I (BMI = 30.0–34.9 kg/m^2), Class II (BMI = 35.0–39.9 kg/m^2) and Class III (BMI ≥ 40 kg/m^2). These values were not chosen arbitrarily; they were based on increases in morbidity as well as mortality at various levels of BMI (2). Adverse effects are observed to some extent between BMIs of 25 and 30 kg/m^2 for some conditions, and more dramatically after a BMI of 30 kg/m^2 (14). Because the distribution of excess body fat is an important modifier of risk (13,14), waist circumference is taken into consideration as an additional criterion to BMI in assessing health risk, as shown in Table 1-2. In the case of abdominal fat deposition, even mild excess adiposity may pose a medical problem. This is especially true for levels of overweight and obesity below Class II (2). As BMI increases beyond 35 kg/m^2, visceral adiposity matters less than the overall impact of the excess adiposity itself. Although a continuum of risk with visceral adiposity exists, a waist circumference of more than 40 inches (102 cm) for men and 35 inches (88 cm) for women have been set as cut-off points for elevated risk (2).

Measurements of body fat percentage as assessed from hydrodensitometry, dual energy X-ray absorptiometry, computed tomography, air displacement plethysmography or other techniques involving multiple-compartment models as criteria to reflect adiposity are generally more accurate, and preferred for metabolic research (15). However, measuring body fat content accurately is too expensive and time-consuming for routine use in clinical practice or population studies. The more common methods that purport to do so, such as use of skinfolds to estimate subcutaneous fat and

Table 1-1A Body Mass Index in Metric Units

Height (cm)	Underweight					Healthy Weight					Overweight					Obesity Class I				
BMI	15	16	17	18	19	20	21	22	23	24	25	26	27	28	29	30	31	32	33	34
								Body Weight (kilograms)												
147.3	32.6	34.7	36.9	39.1	41.2	43.4	45.6	47.7	49.9	52.1	54.3	56.4	58.6	60.8	62.9	65.1	67.3	69.5	71.6	73.8
149.9	33.7	35.9	38.2	40.4	42.7	44.9	47.2	49.4	51.7	53.9	56.1	58.4	60.6	62.9	65.1	67.4	69.6	71.9	74.1	76.4
152.4	34.8	37.2	39.5	41.8	44.1	46.5	48.8	51.1	53.4	55.7	58.1	60.4	62.7	65.0	67.4	69.7	72.0	74.3	76.6	79.0
154.9	36.0	38.4	40.8	43.2	45.6	48.0	50.4	52.8	55.2	57.6	60.0	62.4	64.8	67.2	69.6	72.0	74.4	76.8	79.2	81.6
157.5	37.2	39.7	42.2	44.7	47.1	49.6	52.1	54.6	57.1	59.5	62.0	64.5	67.0	69.5	71.9	74.4	76.9	79.4	81.9	84.3
160	38.4	41.0	43.5	46.1	48.6	51.2	53.8	56.3	58.9	61.4	64.0	66.6	69.1	71.7	74.2	76.8	79.4	81.9	84.5	87.0
162.6	39.7	42.3	44.9	47.6	50.2	52.9	55.5	58.2	60.8	63.5	66.1	68.7	71.4	74.0	76.7	79.3	82.0	84.6	87.2	89.9
165.1	40.9	43.6	46.3	49.1	51.8	54.5	57.2	60.0	62.7	65.4	68.1	70.9	73.6	76.3	79.0	81.8	84.5	87.2	90.0	92.7
167.6	42.1	44.9	47.8	50.6	53.4	56.2	59.0	61.8	64.6	67.4	70.2	73.0	75.8	78.7	81.5	84.3	87.1	89.9	92.7	95.5
170.2	43.5	46.3	49.2	52.1	55.0	57.9	60.8	63.7	66.6	69.5	72.4	75.3	78.2	81.1	84.0	86.9	89.8	92.7	95.6	98.5
172.7	44.7	47.7	50.7	53.7	56.7	59.7	62.6	65.6	68.6	71.6	74.6	77.5	80.5	83.5	86.5	89.5	92.5	95.4	98.4	101.4
175.3	46.1	49.2	52.2	55.3	58.4	61.5	64.5	67.6	70.7	73.8	76.8	79.9	83.0	86.0	89.1	92.2	95.3	98.3	101.4	104.5
177.8	47.4	50.6	53.7	56.9	60.1	63.2	66.4	69.5	72.7	75.9	79.0	82.2	85.4	88.5	91.7	94.8	98.0	101.2	104.3	107.5
180.3	48.8	52.0	55.3	58.5	61.8	65.0	68.3	71.5	74.8	78.0	81.3	84.5	87.8	91.0	94.3	97.5	100.8	104.0	107.3	110.5
182.9	50.2	53.5	56.9	60.2	63.6	66.9	70.3	73.6	76.9	80.3	83.6	87.0	90.3	93.7	97.0	100.4	103.7	107.0	110.4	113.7
185.4	51.6	55.0	58.4	61.9	65.3	68.7	72.2	75.6	79.1	82.5	85.9	89.4	92.8	96.2	99.7	103.1	106.6	110.0	113.4	116.9
188	53.0	56.5	60.1	63.6	67.2	70.7	74.2	77.8	81.3	84.8	88.4	91.9	95.4	99.0	102.5	106.0	109.6	113.1	116.6	120.2
190.5	54.4	58.1	61.7	65.3	69.0	72.6	76.2	79.8	83.5	87.1	90.7	94.4	98.0	101.6	105.2	108.9	112.5	116.1	119.8	123.4
193	55.9	59.6	63.3	67.0	70.8	74.5	78.2	81.9	85.7	89.4	93.1	96.8	100.6	104.3	108.0	111.7	115.5	119.2	122.9	126.6
195.6	57.4	61.2	65.0	68.9	72.7	76.5	80.3	84.2	88.0	91.8	95.6	99.5	103.3	107.1	111.0	114.8	118.6	122.4	126.3	130.1
198.1	58.9	62.8	66.7	70.6	74.6	78.5	82.4	86.3	90.3	94.2	98.1	102.0	106.0	109.9	113.8	117.7	121.7	125.6	129.5	133.4
200.7	60.4	64.4	68.5	72.5	76.5	80.6	84.6	88.6	92.6	96.7	100.7	104.7	108.8	112.8	116.8	120.8	124.9	128.9	132.9	137.0

	Obesity Class II					Obesity Class III														
BMI	35	36	37	38	39	40	41	42	43	44	45	46	47	48	49	50	51	52	53	54
Height (cm)						Body Weight (kilograms)														
147.3	76.0	78.1	80.3	82.5	84.6	86.8	89.0	91.2	93.3	95.5	97.7	99.8	102.0	104.2	106.3	108.5	110.7	112.9	115.0	117.2
149.9	78.6	80.8	83.1	85.3	87.6	89.8	92.1	94.3	96.6	98.8	101.1	103.3	105.6	107.8	110.0	112.3	114.5	116.8	119.0	121.3
152.4	81.3	83.6	85.9	88.3	90.6	92.9	95.2	97.5	99.9	102.2	104.5	106.8	109.2	111.5	113.8	116.1	118.5	120.8	123.1	125.4
154.9	84.0	86.4	88.8	91.2	93.6	96.0	98.4	100.8	103.2	105.6	108.0	110.4	112.8	115.2	117.6	120.0	122.4	124.8	127.2	129.6
157.5	86.8	89.3	91.8	94.3	96.7	99.2	101.7	104.2	106.7	109.1	111.6	114.1	116.6	119.1	121.6	124.0	126.5	129.0	131.5	134.0
160	89.6	92.2	94.7	97.3	99.8	102.4	105.0	107.5	110.1	112.6	115.2	117.8	120.3	122.9	125.4	128.0	130.6	133.1	135.7	138.2
162.6	92.5	95.2	97.8	100.5	103.1	105.8	108.4	111.0	113.7	116.3	119.0	121.6	124.3	126.9	129.5	132.2	134.8	137.5	140.1	142.8
165.1	95.4	98.1	100.9	103.6	106.3	109.0	111.8	114.5	117.2	119.9	122.7	125.4	128.1	130.8	133.6	136.3	139.0	141.7	144.5	147.2
167.6	98.3	101.1	103.9	106.7	109.6	112.4	115.2	118.0	120.8	123.6	126.4	129.2	132.0	134.8	137.6	140.4	143.3	146.1	148.9	151.7
170.2	101.4	104.3	107.2	110.1	113.0	115.9	118.8	121.7	124.6	127.5	130.4	133.3	136.1	139.0	141.9	144.8	147.7	150.6	153.5	156.4
172.7	104.4	107.4	110.4	113.3	116.3	119.3	122.3	125.3	128.2	131.2	134.2	137.2	140.2	143.2	146.1	149.1	152.1	155.1	158.1	161.1
175.3	107.6	110.6	113.7	116.8	119.8	122.9	126.0	129.1	132.1	135.2	138.3	141.4	144.4	147.5	150.6	153.7	156.7	159.8	162.9	165.9
177.8	110.6	113.8	117.0	120.1	123.3	126.5	129.6	132.8	135.9	139.1	142.3	145.4	148.6	151.7	154.9	158.1	161.2	164.4	167.5	170.7
180.3	113.8	117.0	120.3	123.5	126.8	130.0	133.3	136.5	139.8	143.0	146.3	149.5	152.8	156.0	159.3	162.5	165.8	169.0	172.3	175.5
182.9	117.1	120.4	123.8	127.1	130.5	133.8	137.2	140.5	143.8	147.2	150.5	153.9	157.2	160.6	163.9	167.3	170.6	174.0	177.3	180.6
185.4	120.3	123.7	127.2	130.6	134.1	137.5	140.9	144.4	147.8	151.2	154.7	158.1	161.6	165.0	168.4	171.9	175.3	178.7	182.2	185.6
188	123.7	127.2	130.8	134.3	137.8	141.4	144.9	148.4	152.0	155.5	159.0	162.6	166.1	169.7	173.2	176.7	180.3	183.8	187.3	190.9
190.5	127.0	130.6	134.3	137.9	141.5	145.2	148.8	152.4	156.0	159.7	163.3	166.9	170.6	174.2	177.8	181.5	185.1	188.7	192.3	196.0
193	130.4	134.1	137.8	141.5	145.3	149.0	152.7	156.4	160.2	163.9	167.6	171.3	175.1	178.8	182.5	186.2	190.0	193.7	197.4	201.1
195.6	133.9	137.7	141.6	145.4	149.2	153.0	156.9	160.7	164.5	168.3	172.2	176.0	179.8	183.6	187.5	191.3	195.1	198.9	202.8	206.6
198.1	137.4	141.3	145.2	149.1	153.1	157.0	160.9	164.8	168.7	172.7	176.6	180.5	184.4	188.4	192.3	196.2	200.1	204.1	208.0	211.9
200.7	141.0	145.0	149.0	153.1	157.1	161.1	165.2	169.2	173.2	177.2	181.3	185.3	189.3	193.3	197.4	201.4	205.4	209.5	213.5	217.5

Table 1-1B Body Mass Index in Imperial Units

	Underweight					Healthy Weight					Overweight					Obesity Class I				
BMI	15	16	17	18	19	20	21	22	23	24	25	26	27	28	29	30	31	32	33	34
Height (inches)							Body Weight (pounds)													
58	72	77	81	86	91	96	100	105	110	115	120	124	129	134	139	144	148	153	158	163
59	74	79	84	89	94	99	104	109	114	119	124	129	134	139	144	148	153	158	163	168
60	77	82	87	92	97	102	107	113	118	123	128	133	138	143	148	154	159	164	169	174
61	79	85	90	95	101	106	111	116	122	127	132	138	143	148	153	159	164	169	175	180
62	82	87	93	98	104	109	115	120	126	131	137	142	148	153	159	164	169	175	180	186
63	85	90	96	102	107	113	118	124	130	135	141	147	152	158	164	169	175	181	186	192
64	87	93	99	105	111	116	122	128	134	140	146	151	157	163	169	175	181	186	192	198
65	90	96	102	108	114	120	126	132	138	144	150	156	162	168	174	180	186	192	198	204
66	93	99	105	111	118	124	130	136	142	149	155	161	167	173	180	186	192	198	204	211
67	96	102	109	115	121	128	134	140	147	153	160	166	172	179	185	191	198	204	211	217
68	99	105	112	118	125	132	138	145	151	158	164	171	178	184	191	197	204	210	217	224
69	102	108	115	122	129	135	142	149	156	162	169	176	183	190	196	203	210	217	223	230
70	105	111	118	125	132	139	146	153	160	167	174	181	188	195	202	209	216	223	230	237
71	108	115	122	129	136	143	151	158	165	172	179	186	194	201	208	215	222	229	237	244
72	111	118	125	133	140	147	155	162	170	177	184	192	199	206	214	221	229	236	243	251
73	114	121	129	136	144	152	159	167	174	182	189	197	205	212	220	227	235	242	250	258
74	117	125	132	140	148	156	164	171	179	187	195	202	210	218	226	234	241	249	257	265
75	120	128	136	144	152	160	168	176	184	192	200	208	216	224	232	240	248	256	264	272
76	123	131	140	148	156	164	172	181	189	197	205	214	222	230	238	246	255	263	271	279
77	126	135	143	152	160	169	177	185	194	202	211	219	228	236	244	253	261	270	278	287
78	130	138	147	156	165	173	182	190	199	208	216	225	234	242	251	260	268	277	285	294
79	133	142	151	160	169	177	186	195	204	213	222	231	240	248	257	266	275	284	293	302

	Obesity Class II					Obesity Class III															
BMI	35	36	37	38	39	40	41	42	43	44	45	46	47	48	49	50	51	52	53	54
Height (inches)						Body Weight (pounds)															
58	167	172	177	182	187	191	196	201	206	210	215	220	225	230	234	239	244	249	254	258
59	173	178	183	188	193	198	203	208	213	218	223	228	233	238	243	247	252	257	262	267
60	179	184	189	195	200	205	210	215	220	225	230	235	241	246	251	256	261	266	271	276
61	185	190	196	201	206	212	217	222	228	233	238	243	249	254	259	265	270	275	280	286
62	191	197	202	208	213	219	224	230	235	240	246	251	257	262	268	273	279	284	290	295
63	198	203	209	214	220	226	231	237	243	248	254	260	265	271	277	282	288	293	299	305
64	204	210	215	221	227	233	239	245	250	256	262	268	274	280	285	291	297	303	309	315
65	210	216	222	228	234	240	246	252	258	264	270	276	282	288	294	300	306	312	318	324
66	217	223	229	235	242	248	254	260	266	273	279	285	291	297	304	310	316	322	328	334
67	223	230	236	243	249	255	262	268	274	281	287	294	300	306	313	319	326	332	338	345
68	230	237	243	250	256	263	270	276	283	289	296	302	309	316	322	329	335	342	348	355
69	237	244	250	257	264	271	278	284	291	298	305	311	318	325	332	338	345	352	359	366
70	244	251	258	265	272	279	286	293	300	307	314	321	327	334	341	348	355	362	369	376
71	251	258	265	272	280	287	294	301	308	315	323	330	337	344	351	358	366	373	380	387
72	258	265	273	280	287	295	302	310	317	324	332	339	346	354	361	369	376	383	391	398
73	265	273	280	288	296	303	311	318	326	333	341	349	356	364	371	379	386	394	402	409
74	273	280	288	296	304	311	319	327	335	343	350	358	366	374	382	389	397	405	413	420
75	280	288	296	304	312	320	328	336	344	352	360	368	376	384	392	400	408	416	424	432
76	287	296	304	312	320	329	337	345	353	361	370	378	386	394	402	411	419	427	435	444
77	295	304	312	320	329	337	346	354	363	371	379	388	396	405	413	422	430	438	447	455
78	303	311	320	329	337	346	355	363	372	381	389	398	407	415	424	433	441	450	459	467
79	311	319	328	337	346	355	364	373	382	390	399	408	417	426	435	444	453	461	470	479

Table 1-2 Classification of Overweight and Obesity by BMI, Waist Circumference and Associated Chronic Disease Risk

		Disease Risk Relative to Normal Weight and Waist Circumference	
Category	BMI (kg/m²)	Men ≤ 102 cm Women ≤ 88 cm	>102 cm >88 cm
Underweight	<18.5	–	–
Normal weight	18.5–24.9	–	–
Overweight	25.0–29.9	Increased	High
Obesity I	30.0–34.9	High	Very high
Obesity II	35.0–39.9	Very high	Very high
Obesity III	>40.0	Extremely high	Extremely high

bioelectrical impedance are often unreliable, have many confounders, and are usually unnecessary in clinical situations.

STATUS OF OBESITY AND WEIGHT MANAGEMENT

The prevalence and severity of obesity in the United States and many other industrialized countries has risen dramatically in the past 20 years. Depending on criteria used, the obese population now represents 20–35% of all adults in the United States (2,4,16,17). Furthermore, obesity among adults has risen 50% in the last 20 years, and 6% from 1998 to 1999 alone (4,17), with increases of as much as 100% in some states (3). These increases are evident in both genders, and across all age, geographic, socioeconomic, and racial ethnic groups in the United States (4).

Although numerous interventions have been shown to help generate weight loss in the short term, few have succeeded in the long term (18–21). This is in spite of a weight loss obsession in the United States, and huge annual expenditures on weight reduction programs and books, diet products and exercise equipment (22–24). The general public is constantly being fed misinformation about solutions to weight control, which leads to prevalent confusion and unhealthful self-initiated approaches to weight loss. Further complicating matters is the proliferation of unsound and ineffective diets (24–26), environmental forces that foster dietary overconsumption and sedentary lifestyles, the ineffectiveness of currently available weight control tools to sustain healthy weights (22), and high rates of recidivism (20). Many obese individuals continue to battle on their own, unaware of resources for permanent healthful weight management.

Despite the adverse health consequences of obesity (see Chapter 7) (2,6,27) and the dramatic increase in its prevalence, obesity treatment is not commonly practised in the primary care setting (22,28). A number of impediments may contribute to physician reluctance to respond to the obesity epidemic as a chronic disease requiring long-term treatment. These impediments include preconceived notions and negative stereotyping regarding obesity (12), the sheer number of obese patients (17), a general lack of background and training in areas of nutrition, physical activity, and obesity management among physicians (29), and difficulties in obtaining reimbursement for treating the condition of obesity (7,30).

CHANGING TRENDS IN OBESITY AND WEIGHT MANAGEMENT

Obesity is gradually gaining recognition as a medical condition requiring long-term or life-long therapy to achieve improved health outcomes (1,2,11). Its multifactorial etiology is known to involve a complex, heterogeneous interplay of genetic, environmental, and behavioral influences (31,32). While much remains to be elucidated regarding the etiology and pathophysiology of obesity, significant advances have occurred in recent decades (31,33–35). As outlined in Table 1-3, key positive developments in the areas of weight management and obesity research include the changing focus of weight control efforts to health outcomes vs. appearance-

Table 1-3 Recent Advances in Weight Management

- Broadening of definitions of success
- Principles for evidence-based weight control techniques
- Multidisciplinary approach
- Individualized care
- Primary prevention
- Emphasis on permanence of change
- Realistic goal setting
- Public health perspectives

oriented goals, and the principles for evidence-based weight control techniques, including individualized, multidisciplinary care (2,11,36). There is increasing stress on the need for primary prevention of weight gain and maintenance of weight loss by a combination of moderation in energy intake and increased energy output, both from a clinical and public health perspective (37). Furthermore, the accumulation of data demonstrating that modest (5–10%) weight reduction results in clinical improvements in several health-related areas should be encouraging to patients, because they need not be as overwhelmed by overly ambitious or unrealistic weight loss goals (38). Although the attainment of weights associated with minimal mortality as the goal may be desirable in the long run, they may be unattainable for many individuals and these new targets may be more realistic (2,36). For some patients, prevention of further weight gain after years of slow, steady increase may be viewed as progress, as well as maintenance of reduced weight, even if it is still within the range of clinically defined obesity (39).

Data collected from individuals successful at weight loss and maintenance have enhanced our understanding of the most effective strategies in the prevention of recidivism, demonstrating the need for permanence of change. Of particular significance are behavioral and attitude adjustments, careful attention to diet and high levels of physical activity (40–42). Encouraging data suggest that behaviors associated with maintenance of weight loss require less effort and become more pleasurable over time (43). In a recent telephone survey, 48% of individuals who had ever lost ≥ 10% of their body weight had maintained this loss for at least 1 year, and 26% had maintained the loss for at least 5 years (44). Although these data are self-reported, they suggest progress in the avoidance of recidivism.

While physician recommendation for lifestyle change has been shown to result in significant health benefits for overweight and obese patients (45,46), most physicians do not routinely make such recommendations (22,28). Proper nutrition, regular physical activity, and behavior modification have all been demonstrated, under proper circumstances, to result in effective weight management (2,10). However, many physicians lack the time, resources, or training to deliver such treatment and to educate and monitor patients effectively with regard to these lifestyle changes. As such, patients may be referred to registered dietitians, exercise physiologists, and specialists in behavior modification to focus on these specific areas of lifestyle management (10). Frequent contact and education from these health professionals during the period of lifestyle adjustment improves patient compliance (2,47,48).

OBESITY AS A MEDICAL CONDITION

Obesity fulfills all of the criteria to be classified as a chronic disease. Usually lasting many years, obesity is progressive and relapsing (11) and is associated with increased health care use and missed days from work (7,49). Through its various impacts on metabolism, morbidity, and mortality, obesity carries multiple adverse health consequences (6,27). As a chronic disease, obesity resembles hypertension, type 2 diabetes, and coronary heart disease (CHD). Just as the therapeutic goal in each of these conditions is to reduce morbidity and mortality, so should it be in obesity (2,6). Recognition of obesity as a chronic disease provides impetus for approaching treatment through a chronic disease model rather than an acute care model. Central to the chronic disease treatment model is a coordinated team of health care professionals who deliver specific therapy in their areas of expertise, and focus on long-term care.

Historically, physicians may not have treated obesity for various reasons. Perhaps physicians underestimate the potential of obesity as increasing risk for morbidity and mortality. However, mounting data point to associations of obesity with a wide spectrum of serious health conditions, as discussed in Chapter 7. A lifestyle consisting of improper diet and sedentary behavior has been cited as the second leading preventable cause of death in the United States, only exceeded by smoking (50). This underscores the critical importance of preventing and treating obesity in the interest of preventing and treating morbidity and mortality (see Chapter 7).

Lack of effective long-term treatments for obesity may promote reluctance on the part of medical care providers to treat obesity in the primary care setting. However, many successful cases of sustained weight loss in previously obese individuals have been documented (40,42), enhancing the understanding of effective strategies in the prevention of recidivism. In a study of individuals who had successfully maintained a weight loss of at least 30 lb for a minimum of 5 years, over 80% had adopted a combination of nutritional, behavioral, and physical activity strategies (40). The development and evaluation of multidisciplinary weight management programs is providing a stronger evidence base for the long-term efficacy of such strategies (10,11,51–53).

Obese patients receiving weight reduction advice from their physicians are significantly more likely to embark on weight loss attempts than those who do not (46,54), yet only an estimated 38% of obese patients are diagnosed as such, and only 42% of obese individuals report weight loss recommendations from their physicians (22). This underscores the need for increased physician involvement in obesity treatment (10,11,55). Promising results have been shown from studies in which physicians have been trained in counseling obese patients (54). In a recent 10-state survey, 77.5% of individuals who had received weight loss advice from a health care practitioner reported weight loss attempts, vs. 33.4% of those who had not received advice (56). National organizations are urging increased involvement on the part of physicians and other health care professionals in obesity treatment and weight management (2,6,36,57).

Lifestyle measures such as improved nutrition, increased physical activity, and behavior modification remain cornerstones in the treatment of obesity. In resistant and severe cases, pharmacotherapy or surgery may be appropriate (2,58). While caloric restriction is a mainstay of obesity therapy, increased physical activity has an important role for both weight loss and the prevention of recidivism. Behavioral modification therapy assists patients as they incorporate these lifestyle changes into their daily lives. Individuals who combine proper nutrition with behavioral strategies and regular exercise have been shown to be significantly more likely to maintain weight loss compared to individuals who simply restrict calories (20,44).

An individualized, multidisciplinary approach has been advocated by national and international organizations focusing on obesity treatment and prevention (1,2,6,36). Such organizations also stress the importance of a health-outcomes focus, realistic goal setting and permanence in lifestyle change. The definition of successful obesity treatment should be broadened to encompass goals other than weight loss. For example, outcomes to target may include improved metabolic profiles, reduced blood pressure or fasting blood lipids and glucose, increased daily physical activity and fitness, greater consumption of fruits, vegetables and fiber, reduction in dietary fat, changes in specific unhealthful habits as well as enhanced self-esteem, self-efficacy, quality of life and functional capacity (2,36,59).

MULTIDISCIPLINARY APPROACHES TO OBESITY TREATMENT

Treatment modalities for effective management of obesity have been extensively investigated for decades. Combination approaches integrating energy intake restriction, increased physical activity and behavior modification have been shown to be the most effective programs for weight loss, weight maintenance and improved quality of life (10). A health care team of professionals in these disciplines provides physicians and patients with the necessary resources to manage a condition that has proven difficult to treat. Multiple health professionals working together as a treatment team have a greater capacity than any one team member alone to enhance the weight management strategies undertaken by the patient, and ultimately improve the patient's health.

According to the treatment algorithm recommended by the NIH (2), 6 months is a reasonable timescale for the initial goal of a 10% reduction in body weight. During this time, strategies should involve dietary energy restriction, increased physical activity, and behavioral modification. After the initial 6 months, maintenance of weight loss is critical and, in some individuals, further weight loss may be attempted if indicated through careful evaluation. The specific weight management strategy should be tailored to meet the individual needs, goals, and circumstances of each patient (2,36).

The growing acceptance of obesity as a chronic disease that should be treated medically may encourage management of obesity in a traditional disease model within the existing health care system (11). Models of multidisciplinary team care offer effective options for continuing long-term management. Such models must provide for medical management of the patient, draw on the resources of nutrition, physical activity, and behavioral counseling, and involve the patient not as a "subject" but as an integral and responsible member of the team. Multidisciplinary team care is frequently applied in the treatment and management of diabetes, cancer, coronary artery disease, and cardiac rehabilitation (12), and its application to obesity care is very appropriate.

The logistics and structure of a multidisciplinary weight management program can vary considerably depending on the time, resources, and circumstances of the physician and other health care practitioners involved. Various models have been described (11,12,52,53), with varying levels of involvement on the part of each team member. For example, if a physician does not have ready access to dietitians, exercise physiologists, and behaviorists, referral may be appropriate. A more integrated structure can be established if a given facility provides an environment for an interactive team. Multidisciplinary models that fall at levels between these two examples may be suited for many facilities (11,12,52).

In multidisciplinary models, the physician may not necessarily "head" or coordinate the team, although in practice the physician often has a key role in motivating obese individuals to undertake and stay with treatment (12). Within the multidisciplinary team model, the physician is usually responsible for providing primary medical assessment and medical management of the patient. Other health professionals on the team can coordinate care among the team members, work with the patient in developing and implementing his or her individual treatment strategy, and provide the ongoing patient support that enhances patient success in reaching and sustaining weight management goals.

It is important that the roles of each team member be clearly defined to assure that all aspects of obesity treatment and weight management are adequately covered for each individual patient, and to avoid redundancy or discrepancies among team members. Examples of appropriate roles for each team member are outlined in Figure 1-1. Some flexibility within these roles may be necessary to accommodate varying needs among individual patients. In this paradigm, the patient is central to the team, with responsibilities for maximizing the efficacy of his or her treatment. As weight management is a lifelong endeavor, it is important that the patient be empowered to manage proactively his or her own weight within the treatment program. Health care professionals can motivate and encourage the patient in this role. Communication between the patient and all the health care professionals is vital, as is communication among the health care professionals. This communication can be achieved through meetings, shared record keeping (written or electronic), telephone calls and the Internet.

The multidisciplinary obesity management team involves integrated efforts by the patient, physician, registered dietitian, exercise physiologist, and behaviorist. Other

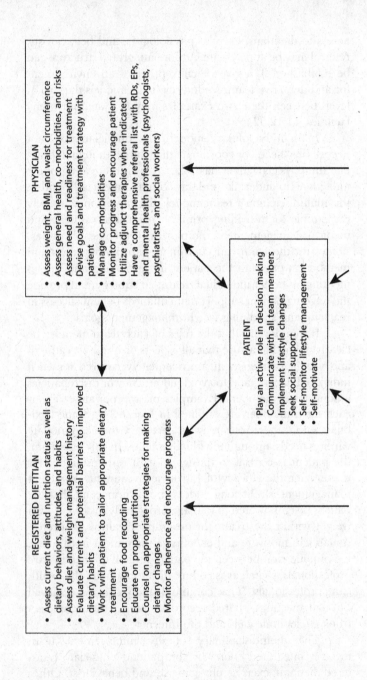

PHYSICIAN

- Assess weight, BMI, and waist circumference
- Assess general health, co-morbidities, and risks
- Assess need and readiness for treatment
- Devise goals and treatment strategy with patient
- Manage co-morbidities
- Monitor progress and encourage patient
- Utilize adjunct therapies when indicated
- Have a comprehensive referral list with RDs, EPs, and mental health professionals (psychologists, psychiatrists, and social workers)

PATIENT

- Play an active role in decision making
- Communicate with all team members
- Implement lifestyle changes
- Seek social support
- Self-monitor lifestyle management
- Self-motivate

REGISTERED DIETITIAN

- Assess current diet and nutrition status as well as dietary behaviors, attitudes, and habits
- Assess diet and weight management history
- Evaluate current and potential barriers to improved dietary habits
- Work with patient to tailor appropriate dietary treatment
- Encourage food recording
- Educate on proper nutrition
- Counsel on appropriate strategies for making dietary changes
- Monitor adherence and encourage progress

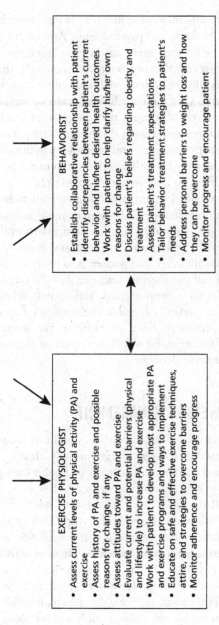

EXERCISE PHYSIOLOGIST

- Assess current levels of physical activity (PA) and exercise
- Assess history of PA and exercise and possible reasons for change, if any
- Assess attitudes toward PA and exercise
- Evaluate current and potential barriers (physical and lifestyle) to increase PA and exercise
- Work with patient to develop most appropriate PA and exercise programs and ways to implement
- Educate on safe and effective exercise techniques, attire, and strategies to overcome barriers
- Monitor adherence and encourage progress

BEHAVIORIST

- Establish collaborative relationship with patient
- Identify discrepancies between patient's current behavior and his/her desired health outcomes
- Work with patient to help clarify his/her own reasons for change
- Discuss patient's beliefs regarding obesity and treatment
- Assess patient's treatment expectations
- Tailor behavior treatment strategies to patient's needs
- Address personal barriers to weight loss and how they can be overcome
- Monitor progress and encourage patient

Figure 1-1 Examples of appropriate roles for members of the multidisciplinary lifestyle weight management team.

team members who may come into play, if indicated, include nurses, social workers, and psychologists. Any health professional on the team may serve as the case manager, as appropriate. However, the physician is frequently the case manager, especially for patients with multiple comorbid conditions. It is vital that the coordinated team of health care professionals is well-organized, non-judgmental toward the patient, encourages progress and motivates the patient in a mutually supportive manner, and promotes positive thinking (36,60). The patient who feels positive about his or her treatment is most likely to adhere and succeed (52).

Careful record keeping and communication are critical in a multidisciplinary weight management team. Intervention strategies need to be documented, status evaluated, progress reviewed, and future directions and goals discussed (36). As a team member, the patient is actively involved in decisions and self-monitoring, and can have a crucial role in communication. Computerized, online networking also offers potential, particularly when the team is composed of independent providers. Each provider in the team offers expertise and strategies for a specific aspect of the multidisciplinary treatment of obesity.

LIFESTYLE WEIGHT MANAGEMENT

The multidisciplinary approach to weight management involves the patient making changes in daily lifestyle, under the support and guidance of a team of health care practitioners with various areas of expertise. As discussed earlier, the main goal of the treatment program may not necessarily be focused on decreased body weight, but on changes in medical status, and improvements in lifestyle such as improved nutritional intake, increased physical activity and fitness, and changes in behaviors and attitudes associated with health-related habits. Treatment goals may be more effective when they focus on behavior change, which is under the direct control of the patient, rather than weight loss, which is less directly controlled (60). Therefore, one can view the multidisciplinary treatment program as not necessarily weight management, but lifestyle management. The obese patient learns to manage his or her own lifestyle, leading to improvements in overall health. The team of health care professionals serves to assess and monitor health status and improvements, to provide adjunct therapy if indicated, and to educate, support and encourage the patient as he or she progresses in lifestyle management.

An obesity treatment algorithm has been developed by the NIH, to provide practitioners with a system for decision making in each patient's care (2). The steps of assessment, management and follow-up are outlined in Table 1-4, and referred to in the following sections of this chapter. The NIH document also includes extensive and useful appendices that can be used as patient guidelines, handouts and for self-monitoring (2).

Assessment of the Obese Patient

The medical assessment is an essential first step in treating the obese patient. It is an opportunity for the health care provider to assess the severity and consequences of the obesity in the individual patient, to establish baseline measurements from which change can be detected, and to serve as an instrument for change.

As part of the baseline assessment, the physician should measure the patient's weight, height, BMI, and waist circumference as discussed earlier. Regular waist circumference measurements are recommended in adult patients, because visceral adipose may increase even in the absence of increases in body weight or BMI (13). For waist circumference measurements, it is most appropriate to use bony landmarks, measuring at the mid-distance between the iliac crest and lowest rib (2). The umbilicus may provide an easily determined landmark, but it may move with weight loss or gain, and alignment of the measuring tape across the patient's back may be uncertain, causing difficulty in accurately assessing changes over time. Fortunately, metabolically active abdominal fat is usually very responsive to weight reduction treatments. Initial weight loss will often come from abdominal sources (61). Peripheral body fat is associated with a lesser degree of health risk for a given

Table 1-4 Obesity Assessment and Treatment Guidelines from the National Institutes of Health (NIH)

ASSESSMENT
Measure weight, height and determine BMI
Measure waist circumference
Assess comorbidities
Assess need for treatment
Assess readiness for treatment

MANAGEMENT
Set realistic goals
  Initial weight loss ~10% of body weight over 6 months
  Rate of weight loss ~1–2 lb (0.5–1 kg)/week
Diet
  Energy intake deficit: 500–1000 kcal/day
  Total energy intake never below 800 kcal/day
Physical activity
  Gradually work toward >30 min moderate-intensity
    physical activity on most, and preferably all, days of
    the week
Behavior
  Tools include self-monitoring (record keeping), stress
    management, stimulus control, problem solving,
    contingency management, cognitive restructuring, and
    social support

OTHER OPTIONS
Pharmacotherapy
  For eligible high-risk patients, if the patient has not lost
    1 lb/week after 6 months of combined lifestyle therapy
Surgery
  For extreme obesity with comorbidities

ONGOING ASSESSMENT AND FOLLOW-UP
Repeat steps in Assessment above on a regular basis

mass of excess fat, but is less easily modified than centrally distributed fat (13).

The physical examination can yield evidence of possible endocrine factors and detect complicating conditions, which must be taken into consideration in tailoring an individual weight management strategy (62). Laboratory testing can screen for comorbidities and complications of obesity. Blood chemistries should include fasting serum glucose, total lipid profile, and liver tests (2). Blood pressure is very important to measure, and an electrocardiogram is usually desirable. Thyroid-stimulating hormone (TSH-I) levels should be obtained if there is any suspicion of thyroid dysfunction, as well as other endocrine and metabolic tests if there is a specific suspicion. Patients should also be screened for symptoms of sleep apnea and osteoarthritis.

In assessing a patient's overall health status and risk, all of the above measurements (BMI, waist circumference, and comorbid conditions and risk factors) must be taken into account (2). A list of conditions imparting additional risk in obese individuals is presented in Table 1-5. These conditions may act synergistically with obesity in increasing a patient's overall risk, so must be considered in assessment and in determining the aggressiveness of clinical interventions (2).

At baseline, the patient should also be assessed for readiness to change (2,60). Non-physician team members, such as the behaviorist, may perform this if more appropriate. The assessment may include reasons and motivation for weight loss, anticipated social support, understanding of commitment involved, attitudes toward lifestyle changes and potential barriers (59).

The patient's weight history and obesity development may pinpoint precipitants of weight gain and suggest possibilities for treatment. An additionally important consideration is the individual's prior weight loss experiences, which may affect self-efficacy related to modifying eating and exercise behaviors (60). Information on previous weight loss attempts offers insight into reasons why the patient may or may not have been successful, to target specific areas that may be capitalized upon or avoided, respectively (20). Additionally, the history may reveal weight cycling (yo-yo dieting), and behavior disorders such as binge eating, bulimia nervosa or night eating syndrome. When an eating disorder is suspected, merely prescribing a weight loss program may not be helpful and may even be counterproductive. Referral to

Table 1-5 Summary of Conditions Imparting Risk for Morbidity and Mortality in Overweight and Obese Individuals

- Established CHD
- Presence of other atherosclerotic diseases
- Type 2 diabetes
- Sleep apnea
- Cigarette smoking
- High blood pressure: systolic ≥140 mmHg or diastolic ≥90 mmHg
- Serum LDL cholesterol ≥160 mg/dL (borderline–high = 130–159 mg/dL)
- Serum HDL cholesterol ≤35 mg/dL
- Fasting plasma glucose ≥110 mg/dL
- Family history of premature CHD
- Age ≥45 years in men; ≥55 years in women (or postmenopausal)
- Physical inactivity
- Atherogenic lipoprotein phenotype (elevated serum triglycerides, small LDL particles and low HDL levels)
- Elevated hemostatic risk factors

CHD, coronary heart disease; HDL, high-density lipoprotein; LDL, low-density lipoprotein.

a center experienced in the treatment of eating disorders is preferable for such patients. Encouraging the reluctant patient with medical complications of obesity to lose weight is appropriate, but it is also important to recognize that weight loss attempts are likely to fail if the patient is not self-motivated to change (52).

Additional recommended baseline assessments include current dietary intake and patterns, as well as habitual level of physical activity, experience with exercise programs and potential barriers to improving nutrition and physical activity. These assessments may be performed by the registered dietitian and exercise physiologist, respectively, and serve as a basis for the details of the lifestyle management program. From these assessments, a plan can be developed for evaluating the individual's progress along with feedback and reinforcement strategies.

Lifestyle Management for Obese Patients Emphasizing the specific medical reasons and benefits of weight loss, based on initial assessments of an individual, can serve in substantially motivating patients (60). Immediate medical benefits can be expected following even moderate weight loss (5–10%) for most obese individuals (27,63–65) who suffer from clinical complications of obesity (see Chapter 7).

As shown in Table 1-4, after the patient assessment, weight management strategies are designed and implemented. Goal setting should involve all team members, with the patient central to decision making. Goals should be specific, objective, individualized, and realistically tangible (36). For example, the physician may help to set medical goals such as decreasing blood pressure, the dietitian may help set nutritional goals such as reducing portion sizes, the exercise physiologist may help set physical activity goals such as increasing the number of minutes spent walking daily, and the behaviorist may help set behavioral goals such as controlling environmental stimuli.

The approach to the weight loss protocol depends on the degree of obesity (BMI and waist circumference), the presence or absence of comorbidities or conditions imparting increased risk for morbidity and mortality such as those listed in Table 1-5, as well as the results of the behavioral assessment, and the patient's preferences (2). The NIH guidelines for selecting obesity treatment strategies are presented in Table 1-6. For all obese patients, regardless of category, the treatment must emphasize improvements in lifestyle patterns relating to diet, exercise, and behavior. The plan should induce a negative energy balance through both diet and exercise, resulting in a rate of weight loss of 1–2 lb (0.5–1.0 kg) per week. Medication, if prescribed, should be considered as supportive of this primary plan, rather than central. Specific recommendations regarding medications and surgery are presented in Chapters 5 and 6.

Regardless of the specific weight loss plan recommended, it is important to remind the patient that the

Table 1-6 A Guide to Selecting Treatment. (From National Institutes of Health (2) with permission.)

Treatment	BMI Category 25–26.9	27–29.9	30–34.9	35–39.9	≥40
Diet, physical activity, and behavior therapy	With comorbidities	With comorbidities	+	+	+
Pharmacotherapy		With comorbidities	+	+	+
Surgery				With comorbidities	+

Prevention of weight gain with lifestyle therapy is indicated in any patient with a BMI > 25 kg/m², even without comorbidities, while weight loss is not necessarily recommended for those with a BMI of 25–29.9 kg/m² or a high waist circumference, unless they have two or more comorbidities.
Combined therapy with a low calorie diet (LCD), increased physical activity, and behavior therapy provide the most successful intervention for weight loss and weight maintenance.
Consider pharmacotherapy only if patient has not lost 1 lb/week after 6 months of combined lifestyle therapy.
The + represents the use of indicated treatment regardless of comorbidities.

different interventions are only parts of the overall plan and will fail in the long term unless changes in behavior and lifestyle are lasting. The importance of patience and persistence during the gradual process of change in lifestyle and weight should also be emphasized to the patient.

Specific underlying factors that induce a chronically positive energy balance, and thus the development of obesity, differ among individuals, as do daily lifestyle, environment, resources, and social situations (32). As a consequence, not every individual will find that any given approach is appropriate. Therefore, tailoring the treatment to the individual needs of the patient is very important, and has been shown to be effective (2,36,66). The obesity treatment program must be integrated into other aspects of the patient's health care and self-care. Patients should discuss with the appropriate member of the team the approach that best suits their needs. Factors that may make a given strategy most suitable must be considered, including cost, convenience, coexisting health conditions, strategies for adapting to different social situations, and a continued plan for healthful life-long weight maintenance (26). The patient plays a vital part in assuring the integration of lifestyle changes, and communicating with the appropriate members of the multidisciplinary team if problems are encountered in incorporating lifestyle changes into social, cultural, or personal circumstances. The team members can work with the patient in overcoming these challenges as lifestyle improvements are made.

The physician has a key role in this multidisciplinary weight management team, with regular monitoring of patient progress and risk factor status, establishing attainable goals, educating on risk factors associated with excess body weight, encouraging and motivating patients (2,10,11). Some practical guidance that the physician may offer to help patients improve weight management behaviors is listed in Table 1-7.

Important nutritional considerations in planning appropriate diets for weight loss and weight management include the diet's energy content, composition, and suitability for individual patient needs (26). These are discussed in detail in Chapter 3. Food records and checklists are advo-

Table 1-7 Practical Guidance to Help Patients Improve Weight Management Behaviors

- Seek support systems from family, friends, and coworkers
- Keep a simple diary of food intake and physical activities
- Replace energy-dense foods (rich desserts, fried foods, chips, soda) with healthful foods (fruits, vegetables, whole grains, water)
- Substitute sedentary behaviors (e.g. television viewing) with more active behaviors (e.g. going for a walk)
- If viewing television, avoid using a remote control and eating
- Park car farther away from stores, work, etc.
- Take the stairs instead of the elevator

cated as excellent tools for increasing patient awareness of energy and nutrient intakes, monitoring of progress, and discussing appropriate adjustments with the dietitian (51).

All recommendations for physical activity should be based on the medical evaluation and take into account any coexisting medical conditions. Individual activity programs for obese patients should ideally include aerobic activity and exercise, stretching, strength (resistance) training, and increased daily lifestyle activities (67). Whatever the scope of the physical activity program, aerobic exercise should be the primary "formal" exercise program. Exercise and physical activity strategies in obesity treatment and management are discussed in detail in Chapter 2. Self-monitoring tools such as activity diaries, patient education resources, and support follow-up from the health care team (in the form of phone, e-mail or consultation) can improve long-term adherence to the patient's physical activity and total weight management program.

Although research into the relationship of energy intake, physical activity and weight management has led to the development of specific dietary and activity guidelines, simply increasing a patient's knowledge regarding the most appropriate levels of dietary intake and physical activity for weight management may be ineffective unless supported by a strong behavioral component (51). By working with a specialist in behavior modification, patients can systematically target specific behaviors and attitudes that potentiate their obesity, and develop tailored strategies to change them and overcome barriers to weight loss. Details on effective behavioral approaches in weight management are presented in Chapter 4.

Ongoing Assessment and Follow-up Weight, BMI and waist circumference should be measured on a regular basis as the lifestyle management program progresses, even if weight change is not the primary outcome of interest (2). Sustained rates of weight loss that are too rapid or too slow may indicate that the prescribed levels of energy intake and/or expenditure may be inappropriately balanced. Ongoing integration of the dietary plan with physical activity recommendations and behavioral modification support is critical throughout a weight management program. This underscores the importance of communication among team members. If the rate of weight loss is slow and inconsistent, the patient should not be discouraged, especially if lifestyle and health improvements are progressing. The patient should be reminded that moderate decreases in body weight, as well as improved diet and physical activity, have been associated with significant improvements in health status and quality of life (38,68). Thus, modest weight loss should not be considered a failure or a waste of time, and can be used to provide encouragement, positive feedback, and reinforcement for the patient.

Regular visits to weigh patients, encourage them, review adherence, and discuss future progress have been associated with improvements in weight loss (2,51). Such visits may be brief and may be conducted by any member of the multidisciplinary team, and should also include measurements of blood pressure and pulse. Any improvements in health status should be shared with the patient as a means of encouragement and reinforcement. In general, it is best to schedule visits most frequently at the start of the program, for example, every 1–4 weeks, in order to monitor the treatment's effectiveness and potential side-effects. After 3–6 months, the visits can become less frequent as the patient becomes more independent in lifestyle weight management. The appropriate frequency of visits and duration of treatment should be carefully discussed among all team members, including the patient. Both increased visit frequency and longer treatment duration have been positively correlated with successful outcomes (2,21,47), although the effective visit can be rather brief (<15 min) (51). Promising results have also been reported from programs utilizing web-based contact for ongoing follow-up (69).

Patient contact with health care professionals is an important consideration in developing and implementing lifestyle interventions for obesity treatment. For the patient, maintaining contact with a structured treatment program is one of the strongest determinants of long-term weight loss (51). Frequent contact and education from health professionals during the period of lifestyle adjustment improves patient compliance (2). Implementation of a high-contact intervention program may include integrating the primary care setting, clinical programs, group-delivered education, and mediated approaches such as postal mail, telephone, and the Internet.

Throughout the lifestyle weight management program, strategies for permanence of change should be integrated, so that the patient can become increasingly self-sufficient. The importance of enduring improvements in diet, physical activity, and behavior must be emphasized to assure long-term maintenance of a healthier weight, and to prevent recidivism. Long-term weight maintenance should be viewed as an ongoing process rather than a last step in a behavior change program (70,71).

CONCLUSIONS

Multidisciplinary lifestyle weight management involves the obese patient learning to manage his or her own lifestyle, leading to improvements in overall health. The patient is supported by a team of health care professionals serving to assess and monitor health status and improvements, to provide adjunct therapy if indicated, and to educate, guide, and encourage the patient as he or she progresses in lifestyle management. The ultimate outcomes are long-term changes in lifestyle that lead to permanent improvements in health and quality of life. By drawing on the combined resources of the physician and other health care professionals with expertise in the treatment of obesity, and by working with the obese patient as an actively involved member of the team, the multidisciplinary approach to managing obesity offers promise of flexible, individualized, and effective strategies for enduring lifestyle weight management.

REFERENCES

1. World Health Organization. Obesity: preventing and managing the global epidemic. Report of a WHO Consultation presented at the World Health Organization; June 3–5, 1997; Geneva Switzerland. Publication WHO/NUT/NCD/98.1.
2. National Institutes of Health. Clinical guidelines on the identification, evaluation, and treatment of overweight and obesity in adults: the evidence report. Bethesda, MD: National Heart, Lung and Blood Institute; June 1998.
3. Mokdad AH, Serdula MK, Dietz WH, Bowman BA, Marks JS, Koplan JP. The spread of the obesity epidemic in the United States, 1991–1998. JAMA 1999; 282: 1519–1522.
4. Mokdad AH, Serdula MK, Dietz WH, Bowman BA, Marks JS, Koplan JP. The continuing epidemic of obesity in the United States. JAMA 2000; 284: 1650–1651.
5. Must A, Spandano J, Coakley EH, Feild A, Colditz G, Dietz W. The disease burden associated with overweight and obesity. JAMA 1999; 282: 1523–1529.
6. National Task Force on the Prevention and Treatment of Obesity. Arch Intern Med 2000; 160: 898–904.
7. Wolf AM, Colditz GA. Current estimates of the economic cost of obesity in the United States. Obes Res 1998; 6: 97–106.
8. Fine JT, Colditz GA, Coakley EH, Moseley G, Manson JE, Willett WC, Kawachi I. A prospective study of weight changes and health-related quality of life in women. JAMA 1999; 282: 2136–2142.
9. Ford ES, Moriarty DH, Zack MM, Mokdad AH, Chapman DP. Self-reported body mass index and health-related quality of

life: findings from the behavioral risk factor surveillance system. Obes Res 2001; 9: 21–31.

10. Rippe JM. The obesity epidemic: a mandate for a multidisciplinary approach. J Am Diet Assoc 1998; 98 (10): S1–S64.

11. Hill JO. Dealing with obesity as a chronic disease. Obes Res 1998; 6 (suppl 1): 34–38.

12. Frank A. A multidisciplinary approach to obesity management: the physician's role and team care alternatives. J Am Diet Assoc 1998; 98 (suppl 2): 44–48.

13. Després J-P. The insulin resistance–dyslipidemic syndrome of visceral obesity: effect on patients' risk. Obes Res 1998; 6 (suppl 1): 8–17.

14. Willett WC, Dietz WH, Colditz GA. Guidelines for healthy weight. N Engl J Med 1999; 341: 427–434.

15. Ellis KJ. Human body composition: in vivo methods. Physiol Rev 2000; 80: 649–680.

16. Kuczmarski RJ, Flegal KM, Campbell SM, Johnson CL. Increasing prevalence of overweight among US adults: the National Health and Nutrition Examination Surveys, 1960–1991. JAMA 1994; 272: 205–211.

17. Flegal KM, Carroll MD, Kuczmarski CJ, Johnson CL. Overweight and obesity in the United States: prevalence and trends, 1960–1994. Int J Obes 1998; 22: 39–47.

18. Sayer D. Diet, behavior modification, and exercise: a review of obesity treatments from a long-term perspective. South Med J 1991; 84: 1470–1474.

19. Wadden TA. The treatment of obesity: an overview. In: Stunkard AJ, Wadden, eds. Obesity: theory and therapy. New York: Raven Press, 1993: 197–217.

20. Pasman WJ, Saris WHM, Westerterp-Plantenga MS. Predictors of weight maintenance. Obes Res 1999; 7: 43–50.

21. Jeffery RW, Drewnowski A, Epstein LH, Stunkard AJ, Wilson GT, Wing RR, Hill DR. Long-term maintenance of weight loss: current status. Health Psychol 2000; 19 (suppl 1): 5–16.

22. Galuska DA. Are health care professionals advising obese patients to lose weight? JAMA 1999; 282: 1576–1578.

23. Serdula MK, Mokdad AH, Williamson DF, Galuska DA, Mendlein JM, Heath GW. Prevalence of attempting weight loss and strategies for controlling weight. JAMA 1999; 282: 1353–1358.

24. Allara L. The return of the high-protein, low-carbohydrate diet: weighing the risks. Nutr Clin Pract 2000; 15: 26–29.

25. Dwyer JT, Lu D. Popular diets for weight loss: from nutritionally hazardous to helpful. In: Obesity: theory and therapy, 2nd edn. Stunkard AJ, Wadden TA, eds. New York: Raven Press, 1993: 231–252.

26. Melanson KJ, Dwyer J. Popular diets for treatment of overweight and obesity. In: Handbook of Obesity Treatment.

Wadden TA, Stunkard AJ, eds. New York: Guilford Press, 2002: 249–282.

27. Pi-Sunyer FX. Co-morbidities for overweight and obesity: current evidence and research issues. Med Sci Sports Exerc 1999; 31: S602–S608.

28. Stafford RS, Farhat JH, Misra B, Schoenfeld DA. National patterns of physician activities related to obesity management. Arch Fam Med 2000; 9: 631–638.

29. Wynick M. Nutrition education in medical schools. Am J Clin Nutr 1993; 58: 825–927.

30. Frank A. Conflicts in the care of overweight patients: inconsistent rules and insufficient money. Obes Res 1997; 5: 268–270.

31. Grundy SM. Multifactorial causation of obesity: implications for prevention. Am J Clin Nutr 1998; 67: S563–S572.

32. Borecki IB, Higgins M, Schreiner PJ, Arnett DK, Mayer-Davis E, Hunt SC, Province MA. Evidence for multiple determinants of the body mass index: the National Heart, Lung and Blood Institute Family Heart Study. Obes Res 1998; 6: 107–114.

33. Hill JO, Melanson EL. Overview of the determinants of overweight and obesity: current evidence and research issues. Med Sci Sports Exerc 1999; 31: S515–S521.

34. Yanovski JA, Yanovski SZ. Recent advances in basic obesity research. JAMA 1999; 282: 1504–1506.

35. Pérusse L, Bouchard C. Gene–diet interactions in obesity. Am J Clin Nutr 2000; 72: S1285–S1290.

36. American Dietetic Association. Position of the American Dietetic Association: weight management. J Am Diet Assoc 1997; 97: 71–74.

37. Koplan JP, Dietz WH. Caloric imbalance and public health policy. JAMA 1999; 282: 1579–1581.

38. Goldstein DJ. Beneficial health effects of modest weight loss. Int J Obes Relat Metab Disord 1998; 16: 397–415.

39. Tremblay A, Doucet E, Imbeault P, Mauriège P, Després J-P, Richard D. Metabolic fitness in active reduced-obese individuals. Obes Res 1999; 7: 556–563.

40. Klem M, Wing R, McGuire M, Seagle H, Hill J. A descriptive study of individuals successful at long-term maintenance of substantial weight loss. Am J Clin Nutr 1997; 66: 239–246.

41. Shick SM, Wing RR, Klem ML, McGuire MT, Hill JO, Seagle H. Persons successful at long-term weight loss and maintenance continue to consume a low-energy, low-fat diet. J Am Diet Assoc 1998; 98: 408–413.

42. McGuire MT, Wing RR, Klem ML, Hill JO. Behavioral strategies of individuals who have maintained long-term weight losses. Obes Res 1999; 7: 334–341.

43. Klem ML, Wing RR, Lang W, McGuire MT, Hill JO. Does

weight loss maintenance become easier over time? Obes Res
2000; 8: 438–444.

44. McGuire MT, Wing RR, Hill JO. The prevalence of weight loss
maintenance among American adults. Int J Obes Relat Metab
Disord 1999; 23: 1313–1319.

45. Bull FC, Jamrozik K. Advice on exercise from a family physician can help sedentary patients to become active. Am J Prev
Med 1998; 15: 85–94.

46. Kreuter MW, Chheda SG, Bull FC. How does physician advice
influence patient behavior?: evidence for a priming effect.
Arch Fam Med 2000; 9: 426–433.

47. Perri MG, Sears SF Jr, Clark JE. Strategies for improving
maintenance of weight loss: toward a continuous care model
of obesity management. Diabetes Care 1993; 16: 100–109.

48. Wadden TA, Berkowitz RI, Vogt RA, et al. Lifestyle modification in the pharmacologic treatment of obesity: a pilot investigation of a primary care approach. Obes Res 1997; 5:
218–226.

49. Burton WN, Chen C-Y, Schultz AB, Edington DE. The economic costs associated with body mass index in the workplace. J Occup Environ Med 1998; 40: 786–792.

50. McGinnis JM, Foege WH. Actual causes of death in the
United States. JAMA 1993; 270: 2207–2212.

51. Wadden TA, Vogt RA, Andersen RE, Bartlett SJ, Foster GD,
Kuehnel RH, et al. Exercise in the treatment of obesity:
effects of four interventions on body composition, resting
energy expenditure, appetite, and mood. J Consult Clin
Psychol 1997; 65: 269–277.

52. Kushner R, Pendarvis L. An integrated approach to obesity
care. Nutr Clin Care 1999; 2: 285–291.

53. Senekal M, Albertse EC, Momberg DJ, Groenewald CJ, Visser
EM. A multidimensional weight-management program for
women. JAMA 1999; 99: 1257–1264.

54. Simkin-Silverman LR, Wing RR. Management of obesity in
primary care. Obes Res 1997; 5: 603–612.

55. Rippe JM. The case for medical management of obesity: a
call for increased physician involvement. Obes Res 1998;
suppl 1: 23–33.

56. Sciamanna CN, Tate DF, Lang W, Wing RR. Who reports
receiving advice to lose weight?: results from a multistate
survey. Arch Intern Med 2000; 160: 2334–2339.

57. Eckel R. Obesity and heart disease: a statement for the
healthcare professionals from the Nutrition Committee,
American Heart Association. Circulation 1997; 96:
3248–3250.

58. Poston WSC, Foreyt JP. Successful management of the obese
patient. Am Fam Physician 2000; 61: 3615–3622.

59. Foreyt JP, Poston WSC. The role of the behavioral counselor

in obesity treatment. J Am Diet Assoc 1998; 98 (suppl 2): 27–30.

60. Clark MM, Pera V, Goldstein MG, Thebarge RW, Guise BJ. Counseling strategies for obese patients. Am J Prev Med 1996; 12: 266–270.

61. Ross R, Rissanen J. Mobilization of visceral and subcutaneous adipose tissue in response to energy restriction and exercise. Am J Clin Nutr 1994; 60: 695–703.

62. Franz MJ. Managing obesity in patients with comorbidities. J Am Diet Assoc 1998; 98 (suppl 2): 39–43.

63. Reaven GM, and staff of the Palo Alto GRECC Aging Study Unit. Beneficial effect of moderate weight loss in older patients with non-insulin-dependent diabetes mellitus poorly controlled with insulin. J Am Geriatr Soc 1985; 33: 93–95.

64. Wing RR, Koeske R, Epstein LH, Nowalk MP, Gooding W, Becker D. Long-term effects of modest weight loss in type 2 diabetic patients. Arch Intern Med 1987; 147: 1749–1753.

65. Van Gaal LF, Wauters MA, De Leeus IH. The beneficial effect of modest weight loss on cardiovascular risk factors. Int J Obes 1997; 21: S5–S9.

66. Feuerstein M, Papciak A, Shapiro S, Tannenbaum S. The weight loss profile: a biopsychosocial approach to weight loss. Int J Psychiatry Med 1989; 19: 181–192.

67. McInnis KJ. Exercise and obesity. Coron Artery Dis 2000; 11: 111–116.

68. Rippe JM, Price JM, Hess SA, Kline G, DeMers KA, Damitz S, Kreidieh I, Freedson P. Improved psychological well-being, quality of life and health practices in moderately overweight women participating in a 12-week structured weight loss program. Obes Res 1998; 6: 208–218.

69. Tate DF, Wing RR, Winett RA. Using internet technology to deliver a behavioral weight loss program. JAMA 2001; 285: 1172–1177.

70. Wing RR. Cross-cutting themes in maintenance of behavior change. Health Psychol 2000; 19 (suppl 1): 84–88.

71. Vansant G, Hulens M, van der Borgth W, Demyttenaere K, Lysens R, Muls E. A multidisciplinary approach to the treatment of obesity. Int J Obes Relat Metab Disord 1999; 23 (suppl 1): 65–68.

Chapter 2

Exercise Management of the Obese Patient

David Neubauer Lombard and
Tamara Neubauer Lombard

Even given decades of research, weight management is still a matter of creating a deficit between caloric intake and energy expenditure. Is decreasing caloric intake the most appropriate goal for weight reduction programs? Population studies would suggest not. In both the United States and Europe, population surveys indicated that over the past several decades the average daily caloric intake has been decreasing, yet the average weight and rates of obesity have been increasing (1). This has led to the conclusion that energy expenditure, not caloric intake, should be the focus for successful weight loss efforts (2).

Past research indicates physical activity is the single most important behavior for long-term weight management in obese people (3,4). Many controlled trials demonstrate that individuals who are physically active lose more weight than non-active individuals. Moreover, individuals who maintain weight loss typically report exercising regularly vs. those who do not maintain their weight loss (5,6). Physical activity produces behavioral, psychological, and physiological effects, which facilitate weight loss and the ultimate maintenance of weight loss (7–9). This chapter briefly examines the physiological effects of physical activity, which promotes weight loss and weight maintenance, and then presents the difficulty in initiating and maintaining a physical activity program. A brief review of strategies shown to be helpful in maintaining physical activity is presented.

ENERGY EXPENDITURE

Physical activity is the most easily controllable way to increase energy expenditure. Daily bouts of physical exercise increase the energy expenditure by the number of calories needed to perform the chosen activity. Simple, but is there an optimal amount or intensity of exercise? The American College of Sports Medicine (ACSM) has set guidelines for recommended physical activity of 30 min, three times per week, at 70% of capacity (10). However, it must be remembered that the ACSM guidelines are for aerobic fitness, not weight loss. For weight loss, there is the need to create a calorie deficit each day, not just 3 days per week. The greater the deficit, the greater the weight loss. Kelly Brownell (11) and others have recommended daily bouts of physical activity of up to 60 min to create continuous weight loss through daily deficits between energy intake and energy expenditure.

Energy Expenditure During Physical Activity

If daily bouts of physical exercise are optimal, then at what level of intensity should the activity be done? Should exercise be performed at a low intensity over a long duration to burn numerous calories without much stress on the body (10)? Alternatively, should exercise be performed at a high intensity for a short duration (12)? Research indicates that higher intensity exercise shows a greater decrease in subcutaneous skinfolds compared to low-intensity exercise even when total energy expenditure is controlled (13).

What are the factors that influence energy expenditure during exercise and why would higher intensity exercise be more successful in decreasing weight? Several factors influence energy expenditure during physical activity. First, the total amount of work performed. For example, running 5 miles requires five times the work to run 1 mile if the running pace is the same. Energy expenditure is a fairly linear relationship as long as the task performed is at the same intensity. Secondly, the efficiency of work can greatly influence energy expenditure. As intensity of the activity performed increases, there appears to be a decrease in the efficiency of the human body to perform the activity. This reduction in efficiency has been shown in cycling (14–16), walking (17), and weight training (18–20). For example, 22% more energy is required to cycle at high intensity vs. low intensity for the same distance (16). Also, 200% more energy is required for one bench press at 80% of maximum vs. four bench presses at 20% of maximum (18).

Why do we see this relationship between increased intensity of activity causing decreases in work efficiency and thus greater energy expenditure? There are numerous theories. First, as intensity increases there is an increased dependence on the inefficient fast twitch muscle fibers (21), an increase in recruitment of the heart and respiratory muscles (18), and increased recruitment of stabilizing muscles (18). Secondly, as intensity increases there is increased energy expenditure required to remove excess lactate. Thirdly, the changes in the myosis of adenosine triphosphatase (ATPase) activity to cross-bridge sweep ratio and sympathetic nervous activity (12). Regardless of which factors most impact why we see this change in energy expenditure, at higher volumes of high-intensity exercise there will be the greatest effect in increasing energy expenditure during physical activity. Unfortunately, high-intensity high-volume exercise is very fatiguing, has increased risk for injury, and has a low patient compliance rate. Therefore, we recommend use of interval training; a mixture of high and moderate intensity time periods within the workout session.

Resting Energy Expenditure

Increased energy expenditure during activity is only one target for weight management. A second target is to increase resting energy expenditure. For decades people have attempted to increase their resting energy expenditure with the use of stimulants and other very questionable supplements. Recent research has suggested increasing the frequency of intense exercise bouts may be the optimal natural process for increasing resting energy expenditure.

What impact does an individual exercise session have on resting energy expenditure? There is a 5–15% increase in resting energy expenditure for 1–2 days post aerobic exercise of at least 70% of $V_{O_{2max}}$, but not for lower levels of physical activity (16,22–24). Athletes have approximately 5–20% higher resting energy expenditure compared to sedentary controls even after controlling for total body fat (25). These studies suggest high-intensity exercise will not only increase energy expenditure during the exercise bout, but will also continue creating a calorie deficit for up to 2 days by increasing the energy the body uses when at rest.

Why is there this observed increase in resting energy expenditure? One theory is that the increase in muscle mass is the cause, but there is little increase in muscle mass for each acute episode of exercise. Therefore this theory is unlikely to be true. Another theory is driven by the fact there are increases in serum norepinephrine levels following high-intensity aerobic exercise for up to 24 h (22). This increase in norepinephrine and the increase in sympathetic tone may be partially responsible for the observed exercise-induced increase in resting energy expenditure. Whatever the reason, high-intensity exercise can increase the body's resting energy expenditure up to 200 kcal/day for 48 h (12).

As yet research has examined only aerobic exercise, not weight training. Increasing muscle mass or fat-free mass requires high-intensity training. Weight training is generally done as a high-intensity exercise over a short duration to increase fat-free muscle mass and to increase energy expenditure, but we also see subsequent increases in resting energy expenditure. Professional body builders have resting energy expenditures up to 30% higher than controls (12). Even amateur weight trainers have 5–15% higher resting energy expenditure compared to controls (26–29). These findings are independent of the increase in resting energy expenditure for 1–2 days after each acute episode of exercise (12,30).

Given all the correlated findings above, what can we actually say about physical activity as well as the intensity of the activity and its relationship with realized weight loss? Several studies have shown that high-intensity exercise is inversely related to rates of obesity (31–33) and lower waist:hip ratios (34). Furthermore, high-intensity exercise is independently and negatively related to weight gain on 2-year follow-up after initial weight loss (32). However, the problem remains that many people do not like engaging in high-intensity exercise, in some cases because of low baseline fitness levels (35). Perhaps the best recommendation is for a combination of daily moderate-intensity exercise to increase daily expenditure of energy with semi-daily episodes of higher intensity exercise to increase optimal energy expenditure.

AEROBIC EXERCISE IMPACT ON CALORIC INTAKE

Given the recommendations for increased energy expenditure through physical activity, should there be the concern of possible increased calorie consumption secondary to the increased activity levels? Recent reviews by Perri (36) suggested low to moderate levels of exercise are not associated with increases in appetite. Further, Wood et al (37) found moderate exercise might limit preference for dietary fat. What about higher intensity exercise?

One theory suggests that there is an exercise-induced suppression of energy intake/hunger (38–40). Kissileff et al (41) had two groups each of obese and non-obese subjects exercise at either a strenuous or a moderate level. After each acute bout of exercise, the subjects were offered food to eat. The researchers found no difference in the amount of food eaten for the obese subjects. However, in the non-obese groups, those who engaged in high-intensity exercise ate less than those in the moderate level of exercise group. Kissileff et al's (41) results suggest that obese subjects may have a psychological nature that overrides the exercise-induced suppression of appetite.

Although this study found changes in food consumed, most others have only found decreases in reported hunger after high-intensity exercise, but not for actual caloric intake

(42). Still others (38,39,43,44) report suppression of hunger immediately following bouts of intense exercise. Why do we see this decrease? Theories include elevations in body temperature (45), increases in levels of lactic acid (46), and increases in tumor-necrosing factor (47). Regardless of why this difference occurs, the suppression of appetite is short-acting and may not actually decrease overall daily caloric intake.

Does how long one waits to eat after an exercise session have an impact on calorie consumption? Verger et al (48) assessed the impact of offering immediate or delayed meals to subjects after 2 h of physical activity. Food was offered immediately, 1 h, or 2 h after the exercise session. Their results indicated a 2-h delay was related to decreased hunger and calorie intake. Other results confirm the lack of decrease in calorie consumption if one eats too close to the bout of exercise (42,49).

LIFESTYLE ACTIVITY AND CALORIC CONSUMPTION

What impact does lifestyle activity have on calorie consumption? Mayer et al's classic 1956 study of mill workers (50) first found sedentary workers ate as much as the highly active workers, resulting in increased weight. Some cross-sectional studies have found highly active individuals have high intake compared to sedentary individuals but the active individuals tended to be leaner, suggesting a better intake: expenditure ratio (51–53). Hardman (54) also found that highly active subjects had a relatively higher carbohydrate intake. However, others have not found such nutrient-specific selection (51,55).

Numerous longitudinal studies have examined the impact of increased activity on caloric intake. Most studies have revealed no increase in energy intake in response to intervention to increase physical activity (56–59). Dempsy (57) had both obese and non-obese subjects engage in three different physical activity programs with varying intensities. Dempsy found no difference in energy consumption brought about by increased intensity of exercise. Leon et al (58) found no impact on calorie consumption for a 16-week high-intensity walking program. McGowen et al (59) compared the impact of three different intensities of running and found no impact on total caloric intake.

Population, cross-sectional, and longitudinal studies have all suggested that having people increase their physical activity level, even to a high-intensity level, will not create a significant increase in calorie intake. Because food preference may be mostly psychologically and environmentally controlled, dietary choices may be relatively immune to the energy requirements of acute exercise bouts (38–40,60).

DIFFICULTIES IN INITIATING AND MAINTAINING PHYSICAL ACTIVITY

It is clear that physical activity is essential in the management of the obese patient. Fortunately, most individuals in weight-loss programs are successful in initiating exercise programs (8). Unfortunately, just like the non-obese population, individuals who initiate physical activity fail to maintain it over time (10). In addition, while we know that exercising at a greater intensity increases the likelihood of weight loss and the corresponding increases in self-efficacy, we also know that initiating an exercise program at a high intensity for a sedentary population is almost doomed to fail (61). We know that physical inactivity contributes to weight gain, but only 22% of Americans are regularly active (62). Further, methods for maintaining physical activity among the population have shown limited effectiveness (61). Similarly, effective methods for maintaining physical activity in obese individuals are not yet known (8).

Methods showing the most promise in the general population for increasing and maintaining physical activity can be examined for application to the obese population. Fortunately, as noted above, health benefits and weight loss and/or maintenance are associated with moderate-intensity frequent physical activity (i.e. walking, lawn mowing, swimming, housework). This type of activity corresponds well with obese individuals who are likely to be sedentary, may have issues associated with exercising at a high intensity or in public, and who may never have participated in physical activity in their lifetime.

STRATEGIES FOR IMPROVING INITIATION AND MAINTENANCE OF PHYSICAL ACTIVITY

A brief review of the literature reveals behavior change strategies that have been effective in increasing physical activity. These strategies are: self-monitoring, prompting, goal setting, feedback, and problem solving. However, while these strategies have been used to increase initiation of physical activity, they have not shown much effect, if any, on maintenance of physical activity. It is hypothesized that these strategies show potential for maintenance of physical activity when program development combines initiation strategies with those designed for maintenance of behavior change.

Prompting

Kazdin (63) defined prompting as behavior initiation through antecedent events. A prompt is delivered immediately before the opportunity for the behavior. Brownell et al (64) used posted prompts at escalator/stair choice points in a variety of community settings and showed an increase in the use of stairs. After removal of the prompts, the increase in stair use maintained at 1 month, but fell after 3 months. Thus, use of posted prompts showed good effects for initiation if present, but poor continued behavior when removed.

Other researchers have used telephone prompts to increase exercise. Telephone prompts increased attendance and maintenance at a health club (65) and adherence to a home-based program (66). King et al (67) found the addition of weekly phone calls to a home-based intervention had good effects for adoption of physical activity and for fitness levels.

These authors used stimulus control and prompting strategies appropriately for initiation but not for maintenance. Kazdin (63) stated that ideally a program would continue to use the initial cues and then develop other cues to prompt the behavior (e.g. gradually moving toward using environmental or social cues as prompts for the behavior). Importantly, the prompt needs to be specific and within close temporal and spatial proximity to the target behavior. For instance, rather than someone associated with a program calling the exerciser, a friend or spouse could prompt physical activity. A posted cartoon could be used. For example, a cartoon posted on the back of the remote control, on the television dial, on the refrigerator, or on the dashboard of the car could prompt physical activity at an activity/ sedentary choice point. Thus, prompting could potentially be effective for maintenance of physical activity.

Goal Setting

Kazdin (63) defined goal setting as specification of a behavior or set of behaviors to be performed at a specified period of time. Bandura (68) stated goal setting is most effective when individuals set challenging but achievable goals.

Through several studies, Martin et al (69) assessed the differential effects of individual goal setting. One study examined the effect of distance goals (i.e. distance to walk) vs. time goals (i.e. time to walk). Adherence required class attendance plus a third day run outside of class. Results show greater adherence for time goals (76.4%) than for distance goals (67.3%). At 3-month follow-up, time goals and distance goals showed similar maintenance (23 vs. 29%).

The next study examined distance goals—because they were more convenient to administer—within a fixed goal (i.e. consistent goal over time) or a flexible goal condition (i.e. goal changes over time). Flexible goal setting showed a greater effect (83.7%) than fixed goal setting (67.8%). In addition, the flexible goal setting condition showed the lowest dropout rate (0%).

The next study examined the effect of distal (mileage goals set at the beginning and middle of program) vs. proximal (new mileage goals set each week) goal setting with a flexible distance goal. Results indicated greater adherence for the distal goal setting condition (83%) than for the proximal goal setting condition (71%). The investigators found a more pronounced effect at follow-up: distal (67%) and proximal (33%). This result is interesting as behavior modification techniques for initiation stress continual reinforcement and proximal goal setting for continued success. However, this study showed greater short- and long-term effects for a distal goal. Perhaps initiation with distal goals generalized better for longer term adherence than initiation with proximal goals.

Several conclusions can be drawn from the goal setting studies reviewed. First, when individuals set their goals effects are stronger. Secondly, while time goals are effective initially, results do not hold for maintenance. Thirdly, distance goals are more convenient to administer and thus more practical, while showing only slightly less adherence rates than time goals. Fourthly, flexible distal goals show greater initiation and maintenance rates than fixed or proximal goals. Thus, use of goal setting strategies can increase initiation and maintenance rates, but these studies only examined maintenance for 3 months and longer study is necessary for confident conclusions about maintenance.

Feedback

Kazdin (63) defined feedback as information about performance. Feedback is more potent when given for an explicitly defined performance criterion (e.g. physical activity goal). Research shows feedback to be less effective when applied alone than in combination with other reinforcers (63).

Juneau et al (70) provided a portable heart rate monitor that emitted a tone when the exerciser's heart rate increased or decreased from prescribed levels. This home-based program involved self-monitoring of activity levels. Individuals were prescribed exercise 5 days/week. Results showed a fitness increase measured by an increase in Vo_{2max} for both men and women by 12 weeks and continued fitness for 24 weeks. Adherence rates were 90% for men and 75% for women. In addition, they found greater fitness gains corresponded with greater adherence to the program. Another study involving portable heart rate monitors (71) showed Vo_{2max} increases of 14% in men and 10% in women (95%

achieved during the first 12 weeks), with high adherence to the heart rate prescription compared to controls.

These programs involved an explicit performance goal (heart rate prescription) and immediate feedback (when heart rate increased or decreased outside the prescription). This exemplifies an ideal application of feedback. Adherence levels were higher than most studies (e.g. 90 vs. 50%). Unfortunately, the studies provide no follow-up information about maintenance effects.

Martin et al (69) systematically assessed group vs. individual feedback in their series of studies. They encouraged individuals to participate in pairs or small groups. Investigators defined group feedback as information about performance given at the end of a group session and individual feedback as praise twice per exercise session. Individual feedback showed a greater effect on adherence than did group feedback (77.2 vs. 65.8%). At 3-month follow-up both individual and group feedback showed decreased adherence, yet the individual feedback condition decreased significantly less than the group feedback condition (54 and 17%, respectively).

Weber and Wertheim (72) compared three conditions: 1) standard treatment (fitness exam, encouragement and assessment); 2) self-monitoring plus goal setting; and 3) self-monitoring, goal setting plus individual positive feedback. Approximately 78% of participants completed at least 4 weeks of the program in both the self-monitoring and the self-monitoring plus feedback group, with 42% completing at least 10 weeks. Unexpectedly, self-monitoring alone had a greater effect on attendance than self-monitoring plus additional feedback, possibly because additional feedback had no added value on the effect of self-monitoring.

In summary, when feedback was explicit and immediate, adherence was high. Individual feedback showed better initiation and 3-month maintenance effects compared with group feedback. Thus, feedback, when appropriately used and applied with a specific performance criterion (e.g. goal setting), can be effective in increasing and maintaining exercise.

PROBLEM SOLVING TECHNIQUES

Cost–Benefits

Cost–benefit analysis can be defined as any procedure designed to examine the positive and the negative aspects associated with behavior change. Besides the many benefits of exercise (e.g. reduced risk of coronary heart disease, cancer, and obesity) there are many costs to an activity program designed to increase exercise (e.g. sore muscles, time commitment). Often, the costs are much more salient to the individual than the benefits, especially because the costs tend to be encountered immediately, with the benefits far away. Programs typically do not attempt to increase the benefits or decrease the costs associated with physical activity increases. If a program does not fit into an individual's lifestyle, they probably will have difficulty adopting the change and even more difficulty maintaining the change. In addition, Prochaska et al (73) have found that when individuals assess their pros > cons (e.g. benefits greater than costs) they move from contemplation to preparation (i.e. from thinking about performing a behavior to preparing to perform). Some programs have attempted to assess the costs and benefits by use of a decision balance sheet (74,75).

Decision Balance Sheets

The decision balance sheet categorizes anticipated gains (benefits) and anticipated losses (costs) into four major types of consequences:

1. utilitarian gains or losses to self;
2. utilitarian gains or losses for significant others;
3. approval or disapproval from significant others; and
4. self-approval or disapproval (74).

This process involves having individuals consider all information relative to making a decision (e.g. positive consequences, negative consequences), then on a balance sheet grid (with the four headings listed above describing the four major types of decisional consequences) fill in the pros and cons for selected decisions (e.g. time commitment to exercise).

Two of the studies reviewed used decision balance sheets (74,75). Both studies found a significant increase in program adherence when the decision balance sheet was used. The method required little specialized training and only about 20 min per participant. Wankel (76) found decision balance sheets to be effective in a variety of other settings (university-based fitness class, commercial fitness center, and community-based fitness class).

Despite the efficacy of decision balance sheet interventions, some limitations should be noted. First, both studies were less than 2 months in duration and did not allow assessment of effects beyond initial attendance. Thus, while the balance sheet procedure showed initial effects, long-term usage and maintenance effects are unknown. Secondly, the magnitude of the positive effects was not large, perhaps reflecting methodological factors (e.g. definition of adherence, intensity of intervention). Thus, while the decision balance sheet method appeared to have some success, more research is needed to draw definite conclusions.

Other studies attempted to assess costs and benefits by use of problem-solving strategies (77) and identification of costs and benefits (78). Studies using these techniques showed modest increases in physical activity and modest gains in maintenance. The use of problem solving procedures in one study focused these strategies on maintenance (77). This study showed no significant results. Daltroy (78) applied identification of benefits and drawbacks to increase adoption and maintenance and found significant increases in attendance (controlling variables related to the exposure of the intervention). However, investigators showed a 50% dropout by week 12, suggesting that this method may not have adequately addressed maintenance issues.

Thus, when investigators implemented cost–benefit procedures, they showed mixed results. Some showed greater initial adoption with poor maintenance, and others showed little effect. Two issues may explain these inconsistencies. First, cost–benefit analyses performed at the start of a program may be different from analyses performed midway through or after a program. For instance, items or events identified initially as costly may be resolved with new unexpected costs occurring after program initiation (i.e. walking shoes are initially costly, sore muscles and injuries occur later). Secondly, focusing on the initial benefits of exercise may initiate program entry but, once realized, these benefits lose their reinforcing quality. For instance, identifying quick weight loss after initiating regular high-intensity activity may be experienced for a few weeks as a wonderful benefit and a reason to continue exercising. After a few weeks the weight loss may slow and no longer be an identifiable benefit and no longer be reinforcing.

Given its flaws, cost–benefit analyses can still affect increases in physical activity. However, assessment should occur throughout the program to allow for shifts in costs and benefits and to allow for programmed planning to increase the benefits and reduce the costs. Further assessment should continue throughout a program to address maintenance costs and benefits of physical activity.

Self-Monitoring

Most exercise researchers have used some form of self-monitoring strategies to increase exercise adherence. Weber and Wertheim (72) combined self-monitoring with goal setting and feedback and found 78% of participants in a gym setting completed at least 4 weeks of the program. They also found that self-monitoring alone had a greater effect on attendance than self-monitoring plus additional feedback.

Other researchers have found that combining self-monitoring with other behavior change strategies increased physical activity in a variety of settings including: worksite (79); physician's office (80); home-based (67); and cardiac rehabilitation programs (81). Thus, self-monitoring is shown to be a simple and effective strategy to increase physical activity. However, no effects for maintenance of activity are noted.

Maintenance

Initiation/adoption of physical activity through behavioral or cognitive behavioral strategies has shown good results

(69,74,80,82,83). However, maintenance of this behavior change has shown poor results (69,77,84). When physical activity promotion programs are examined it is apparent that they are designed to increase rather than maintain activity as the strategies used are designed for initiation rather than maintenance (e.g. frequent reinforcement, continual feedback). Kazdin (63) suggested response maintenance and transfer of training as appropriate strategies for maintenance. He defined response maintenance as the extension of behavior change over time, and transfer of training as the extension of behavior change to new situations and new settings. Unfortunately, response maintenance and transfer of training are not often used in physical activity promotion programs.

One strategy to promote maintenance is gradually removing or fading the contingencies. Ideally, withdrawing reinforcers gradually leads to complete elimination of the initial reinforcer without a return of behavior change to baseline (63). For example, an individual who is vacuuming for exercise and receiving an encouraging phone call each week initially, then receives a phone call biweekly, then once a month, bi-monthly, once a year, then no phone calls, but continues to exercise. This procedure prepares participants for normal conditions (i.e. conditions under which they must normally perform the behavior).

Use of self-control procedures and cognitively-based procedures are also potential maintenance strategies. Kazdin (63) stated that self-control training involves teaching individuals to control their own behavior through the use of self-reinforcement, self-monitoring, and self-evaluation (alone or together). This training aids in the transition from externally managed programs to environmentally managed programs. Kazdin (63) defined cognitively-based procedures as self-instruction training and problem solving skills training: specialized forms of self-control strategies. Developing self-control strategies allows individuals to develop skills that can be applied across settings and situations. For example, walking program participants can be taught to self-monitor their walking, reward themselves frequently initially, and then fade their reinforcement over time, based on self-evaluation (e.g. goal-setting and feedback). In addition, participants can be taught to generate problem situations (e.g. walking while on vacation or while the children are sick), plan a solution and then practise carrying out the plan (e.g. walk while on vacation). These strategies have been found to be effective in maintaining both a walking program (85) and a lifestyle physical activity program (86).

Lifestyle Physical Activity

One of the most important decisions in conducting physical activity research is what type of physical activity to promote. Some of the barriers to performing physical activity are the perceived discomfort of the activity, the time allowed for activity, and access to facilities (87). As such, individuals should be allowed to choose the activity they feel "fits best" with their lifestyle. Recent studies suggest the activity need not be what individuals typically think constitutes exercise (e.g. jogging, aerobics classes, Stairmasters). Rather, lifestyle activities such as gardening, vacuuming, walking, and choosing stairs over the elevator can result in health-related improvements if performed consistently over time. In fact, it may prove easier to maintain an activity that "fits" into one's lifestyle, rather than an activity that requires an individual to "make time". Thus, individuals should choose the activity they believe they can perform over time (i.e. self-efficacy), that they will enjoy, and that can produce health benefits if performed consistently over time.

The Centers for Disease Control and Prevention recently published a report emphasizing the importance and the health benefits achieved by lifestyle activity (10). In addition, Rippe et al (88) reviewed the physical and psychological benefits of low to moderate intensity exercise. They found that physical activity at this level had several health benefits including: decrease in cholesterol level (89); control of hypertension through lower blood pressure (90); increases in Vo_{2max} (91); control of weight loss through decreased appetite (92); and increases in overall mood state (93). Furthermore, Rippe et al (87) indicated that walking is an ideal target behavior for people with varying medical conditions including: diabetes (94); pregnancy (95); and cardiac rehabilitation (92). More recent studies have directly compared the effects of lifestyle activity vs. structured activity on factors such as weight, body composition, and cardiovascular profiles (96,97). Dunn et al (96), in their 2-year randomized trial comparing effects of lifestyle physical activity and traditional structured exercise with over 200 healthy inactive, somewhat overweight individuals between the ages of 35 and 60, found improvements in physical activity and cardiorespiratory fitness. Although neither group changed their weight, both groups lowered their body fat. Anderson et al compared 40 obese women between the ages of 21 and 60, again comparing the effects of lifestyle physical activity and structured exercise for 16 weeks with a 1-year follow-up. They found weight loss for both groups, with the lifestyle group regaining less weight at follow-up. Thus, lifestyle activity may offer similar weight loss benefits and perhaps better adherence benefits for obese individuals.

Lifestyle activity has several other benefits for increased maintenance of activity. There can be no cost associated with the individual's choice (e.g. choosing to take the stairs over the elevator, walking, gardening). There is no need for expensive facilities, membership fees, or equipment. In addition, individuals can choose to look for opportunities to engage in lifestyle activity within their day and thus may continue to engage in activity when away from home, away on business, or on vacation. Thus, they have the ability to *maintain* their exercise program even when their schedule or location varies. Further, lifestyle activity allows the individual choice and variety in their activity program which may alleviate some of the boredom of routine programs that correlates with exercise dropout (87).

CONCLUSIONS

Research on the effects of physical activity on obesity has repeatedly shown its benefits, yet the percentage of the United States' population who exercise regularly is very low—approximately 10–20%. A review of the literature indicates that the obese population may respond best to a physical activity program that increases in intensity, recognizes the barriers associated with physical activity and obesity, and which "fits" within the individual's lifestyle. A review of the literature on determinants of exercise suggests that the use of behavior change techniques is important for long-term adherence to physical activity and is therefore associated with greater weight loss maintenance. Furthermore, a review of the behavioral strategies used in the exercise area indicated several conclusions.

1. Telephone prompting can be effective.

2. Individual feedback can also be effective.

3. Goal setting, specifically individualized flexible distal goals, can increase adherence.

4. Self-monitoring can both increase adherence and offer outcome data.

5. Lifestyle activity may relate to long-term maintenance while providing health benefits and maintenance of weight loss.

Thus, a physical activity program incorporating these self-control and prompting strategies with lifestyle activity should be more effective than a program without them.

REFERENCES

1. Heine AF, Weinsier RL. Divergent trends in obesity and fat intake patterns: the American paradox. Am J Med 1997; 102: 259–267.
2. Jeffrey RW, Drewnowski A, Epstein LH, Stunkard AJ, Wilson GT, Wing RR, Hill DR. Long-term maintenance of weight loss: current status. Health Psychol 2000; 19 (suppl 1): 5–16.
3. Foreyt JP, Goodrick K. Do's and don'ts for weight management: exercise is always good, but are some foods bad? Obes Res 1994; 2: 378–379.
4. Pronk NP, Wing RR. Physical activity and long-term maintenance of weight loss. Obes Res 1994; 2: 587–599.
5. Jeffrey RW, Bjornson-Benson WM, Rosenthal BS, et al. Correlates of weight loss and its maintenance over 2 years of follow-up among middle-aged men. Prev Med 1984; 13: 155–168.

6. Kayman S, Bruvold W, Stern JS. Maintenance and relapse after weight loss in women: behavioral aspects. Am J Clin Nutr 1990; 52: 800–807.

7. Bouchard C, Despres JP, Tremblay A. Exercise and obesity. Obes Res 1993; 1: 133–147.

8. Grilo CM, Brownell KD, Stunkard AJ. The metabolic and psychological importance of exercise in weight control. In: Stunkard AJ, Wadden TA, eds. Obesity: theory and therapy. New York: Raven Press, 1993: 253–273.

9. Wadden TA, Vogt RA, Foster GD, Anderson DA. Exercise and the maintenance of weight loss: 1-year follow-up of a controlled clinical trial. J Consult Clin Psychol 1998; 66: 429–433.

10. Pate RR, Pratt M, Blair SN et al. Physical activity and public health: a recommendation from the Centers for Disease Control and Prevention and the American College of Sports Medicine. JAMA 1995; 273: 402–407.

11. Brownell KD. The LEARN Program for weight control. Dallas, TX: American Health, 1998.

12. Hunter GR, Weinsier RL, Bamman MM, et al. A role for high intensity exercise on energy balance and weight control. Int J Obes 1998; 22: 489–493.

13. Tremblay A, Simoneau JA, Bouchard C. Impact of exercise intensity on body fatness and skeletal muscle metabolism. Metabolism 1994; 43: 814–818.

14. Gaeser GA, Brooks GA. Muscular efficiency during steady-rate exercise: effects of speed and work rate. J Appl Physiol 1975; 38: 1132–1139.

15. Gladden LB, Welch HC. Efficiency of anaerobic work. J Appl Physiol 1978; 44: 564–570.

16. Treuth MS, Hunter GR, Williams MJ. Effects of exercise intensity on 24-h energy expenditure/substrate oxidation. Med Sci Sport Exerc 1996; 2: 1138–1143.

17. Donovan CM, Brooks GA. Effects of walking speed and work rate. J Appl Physiol 1977; 43: 431–439.

18. Hunter GR, Belcher LA, Dunnan L, Fleming G. Bench press metabolic rate as a function of exercise intensity. J Appl Sports Sci Res 1988; 2: 1–6.

19. Hunter GR, Kekes-Szabo T, Schnitzler A. Metabolic cost–vertical work relationship during knee extension and knee flexion weight training exercise. J Appl Sport Sci Res 1992; 6: 42–48.

20. Kalb J, Hunter GR. Weight training economy as a function of intensity of the squat and overhead press exercise. J Sports Med Phys Fitness 1991; 31: 154–160.

21. Coyle EF, Sidossis LS, Horowitz JF, Beltz JD. Cycling efficiency is related to the percentage of type I muscle fibers. Med Sci Sports Exerc 1992; 24: 782–788.

22. Poehlman EG, Danforth E. Endurance training increases metabolic rate and norepinephrine appearance rate in older individuals. Am J Physiol 1991; 261: E233–E239.
23. Poehlman EG, Horton ES. The impact of food intake and exercise on energy expenditure. Nutr Rev 1989; 47: 129–137.
24. Poehlman ET, McAuliffe T, Danforth E. Effects of age and level of physical activity on plasma epinephrine kinetics. Am J Physiol 1990; 258: E256–E262.
25. Burke CM, Bullough RC, Melby CL. Resting metabolic rate and postprandial thermogenesis by level of aerobic fitness in young women. Eur J Clin Nutr 1993; 47: 575–585.
26. Treuth MS, Hunter GR, Weinsier RL, Kell SH. Energy expenditure and substrate utilization in older women after strength training: 24-h calorimetry results. J Appl Physiol 1995; 78: 2140–2146.
27. Bosselaers I, Buemann B, Victor OJ, et al. Twenty-four hour energy expenditure and substrate utilization in body builders. Am J Clin Nutr 1994; 59: 10–12.
28. Poehlman ET. A review: exercise and its influence on resting energy metabolism in man. Med Sci Sports Exerc 1989; 21: 515–525.
29. Poehlman ET, Garner AW, Ades PA, et al. Resting energy metabolism and cardiovascular disease risk in resistance and aerobically trained males. Metabolism 1992; 41: 1351–1360.
30. Campbell WW, Crim MC, Young VR, Evans UW. Increased energy requirements and changes in body composition with resistance training in older adults. Am J Clin Nutr 1994; 60: 167–175.
31. DiPietro, Williamson DF, Caspersen DJ, et al. The descriptive epidemiology of selected physical activities and body weight among adults trying to lose weight: the Behavioral Risk Factor Surveillance System Survey. Int J Obes 1989; 17: 69–76.
32. French SA, Jeffery RW, Forster JL, et al. Predictors of weight change over 2 years among a population of working adults: the Healthy Worker Project. Int J Obes 1994; 18: 145–154.
33. Khalidk MEM. The association between strenuous physical activity and obesity in a high and low altitude populations in southern Saudi Arabia. Int J Obes 1995; 19: 776–778.
34. Tremblay A, Despres JP, Leblanc C, et al. Effects of intensity of physical activity on body fatness and fat distribution. Am J Clin Nutr 1990; 51: 153–157.
35. Mattsson E, Larsson UE, Rossner S. Is walking for exercise too exhausting for obese women? Int J Obes 1997; 21: 380–386.
36. Perri MG, Martin D, Leermakers EA, et al. (1997). Effects of

group- versus home-based exercise in the treatment of obesity. J Consult Clin Psychol 65; 278–285.

37. Wood PD, Terry RB, Haskell WL. Metabolism of substrates: diet, lipoprotein metabolism and exercise. Fed Proc 1985; 44: 358–363.

38. King NA, Burley VJ, Blundell JE. Exercise-induced suppression of appetite: effects on food intake and implications for energy balance. Eur J Clin Nutr 1994; 48: 715–724.

39. King NA, Blundell JE. High-fat foods overcome the energy expenditure due to exercise after cycling and running. Eur J Clin Nutr 1995; 49: 114–123.

40. King NA, Blundell JE. Effects of exercise and macronutrient availability on appetite: is there a difference between men and women? Int J Obes 1995; 19 (suppl 4): 91.

41. Kissileff HR, Pi-Sunyer XF, Egal K, et al. Acute effects of exercise on food intake in obese and non-obese women. Am J Clin Nutr 1990; 52: 240–245.

42. Thompson DA, Wolfe LA, Eikelboom R. Acute effects of exercise intensity on appetite in young men. Med Sci Sports Exerc 1988; 20: 222–227.

43. Maxwell BD. Serum free fatty acid concentration during post-exercise recovery. PhD thesis. Tucson, AZ: University of Arizona, 1985.

44. Reger WE, Alison TG. Exercise and appetite. Med Sci Sports Exerc 1987; 19: S38.

45. Andersson B, Larson B. Influence of local temperature changes in the preoptic area and rostral hypothalamus in the regulation of food and water intake. Acta Physiol Scand 1961; 52: 75–89.

46. Baile CA, Zinn WN, Mayer J. Effects of lactate and other metabolites on food intake of monkeys. Am J Physiol 1970; 219: 1606–1613.

47. Grunfield C, Finegold KR. The metabolic effects of tumor necrosis factor and other cytokines. Biotherapy 1991; 3: 143–158.

48. Verger PM, Lanteaume T, Louis-Sylvestre J. Human intake and choice of foods at intervals after exercise. Appetite 1992; 1: 1–7.

49. Schoeller DA. Measurement of energy expenditure in free living human by using doubly labeled water. J Nutr 1988; 11: 1278–1289.

50. Mayer J, Roy P, Mitra KP. Relation between caloric intake, body weight and physical work: studies in an industrial male population in West Bengal. Am J Clin Nutr 1956; 4: 169–175.

51. Blair SN, Ellsworth NM, Haskell WL, et al. Comparison of nutrient intake in middle-aged men and women runners and controls. Med Sci Sports Exerc 1981; 13: 310–315.

52. Maughan RJ, Robertson JD, Bruce AC. Dietary energy and carbohydrate intakes of runners in relation to training load. Proc Nutr Soc 1989; 48: 170A.

53. Richard D. Exercise and the neurobiological control of food intake and energy expenditure. Int J Obes 1995; 19: S73–S79.

54. Hardman AE. Exercise and health. CHO International Dialogue 1991; 2: 1–3.

55. Woo R, Pi-Sunyer FX. Effect of increased physical activity on voluntary intake in lean women. Metabolism 1985; 34: 836–841.

56. Andersson B, Xu M, Rebuffee-Scrive K, et al. The effects of exercise training on body composition and metabolism in men and women. Int J Obes 1991; 15: 75–81.

57. Dempsey JA. Antropometrical measurements on obese and non-obese young men undergoing a program of vigorous physical exercise. Res Q Exerc Sport 1964; 35: 275–287.

58. Leon AS, Conrad J, Hunninghake DB, Serfass R. Effects of a vigorous walking program on body composition and lipid metabolism of obese young men. Am J Clin Nutr 1979; 33: 1776–1787.

59. McGowan CR, Epstein LH, Kupfer DJ, et al. The effects of exercise on non-restricted caloric intake in male joggers. Appetite 1986; 97–105.

60. Reger WE, Allison RA, Kurucz RL. Exercise, post-exercise metabolic rate and appetite. Sports Health Nutr 1986; 2: 117–123.

61. Dishman RK. Exercise adherence: its impact on public health. Champaign, IL: Kinetics Books, 1988.

62. US Department of Health and Human Services. Physical activity and health: a report of the Surgeon General. Atlanta, GA: US Department of Health and Human Services, Centers for Disease Control and Prevention, National Center for Chronic Disease Prevention and Health Promotion, 1996.

63. Kazdin AE. Behavior modification in applied settings. Pacific Grove, CA: Brooks/Cole, 1993.

64. Brownell KD, Stunkard AJ, Albaum JM. Evaluation and modification of exercise patterns in the natural environment. Am J Psychiatry 1980; 137: 1540–1545.

65. Wankel LM, Thompson CE. Motivating people to be physically active: self-persuasion vs. balanced decision-making. J Appl Social Psychol 1977; 7: 332–340.

66. Acquista VW, Wachtel TJ, Gomes CI, et al. Home-based health risk appraisal and screening program. J Commun Health 1988; 13: 43–52.

67. King AC, Taylor CB, Haskell WL, DeBusk RF. Strategies for increasing early adherence to and long-term maintenance of

home-based exercise training in healthy middle-aged men and women. Am J Cardiol 1988; 61: 628–632.

68. Bandura A. Social foundations of thought and action: a social cognitive theory. Englewood Cliffs, NJ: Prentice Hall, 1986.

69. Martin JE, Dubbert PM, Katell AD, et al. Behavioral control of exercise in sedentary adults: studies 1–6. J Consult Clin Psychol 1984; 52: 795–811.

70. Juneau M, Rogers F, DeSantos V, et al. Effectiveness of self-monitored, home-based, moderate intensity exercise training in middle-aged men and women. Am J Cardiol 1987; 60: 66–70.

71. Rogers F, Juneau M, Taylor CB, et al. Assessment by a micro-processor of adherence to home-based moderate-intensity exercise training in healthy, sedentary middle-aged men and women. Am J Cardiol 1987; 60: 71–75.

72. Weber J, Wertheim EH. Relationships of self-monitoring, special attention, body fat percent, and self-motivation to attendance at a community gymnasium. J Sport Exerc Psychol 1989; 11: 105–111.

73. Prochaska JO, Velicer WF, Rossi JS, et al. Stages of change and decisional balance for 12 problem behaviors. Health Psychol 1994; 13: 39–46.

74. Hoyt MF, Janis IL. Increasing adherence to a stressful deci-sion via a motivational balance-sheet procedure: a field experiment. J Personality Social Psychol 1975; 31: 833–839.

75. Wankel LM, Yardley JK, Graham J. The effects of motivational interventions upon the exercise adherence of high and low self-motivated adults. Can J Sports Sci 1985; 10: 147–156.

76. Wankel LM. Decision-making and social support strategies for increasing exercise involvement. J Cardiac Rehabil 1984; 4: 124–135.

77. Meyer AJ, Nash JD, McAlister AL, et al. Skills training in a cardiovascular health education campaign. J Consult Clin Psychol 1980; 48: 129–142.

78. Daltroy LH. Improving cardiac patient adherence to exercise regimens: a clinical trial of health education. J Cardiac Rehabil 1985; 5: 40–49.

79. Durbeck DC, Heinzelman F, Schacter J, et al. The National Aeronautics and Space Administration, US Public Health Service Evaluation and Enhancement program: summary of results. Am J Cardiol 1972; 30: 784–790.

80. Epstein LH, Wing RR. Aerobic exercise and weight. Addict Behav 1980; 5: 371–378.

81. Oldridge NB, Jones NL. Improving patient compliance in cardiac exercise rehabilitation: effects of written agreement and self-monitoring. J Cardiac Rehabil 1983; 3: 257–262.

82. Gettman LR, Ward P, Hagan RD. A comparison of combined

running and weight training with circuit weight training. Med Sci Sports Exerc 1982; 14: 229–234.

83. King AC, Frederiksen LW (1984) Low-cost strategies for increasing exercise behavior: Relapse preparation, training and social support. Behav Modif 1984; 18: 3–21.

84. Reid EL, Morgan RW. Exercise prescription: a clinical trial. Am J Public Health 1979; 69: 591–595.

85. Lombard DN, Lombard TN, Winett RA. Walking to meet health guidelines: the effects of prompting frequency and prompting structure. Health Psychol 1995; 14: 164–170.

86. Lombard TN, Lombard DN, Winett RA. Improving physical activity adherence: the effects of self-control strategies and telephone prompting using lifestyle physical activity. [Dissertation abstract]. Dissertation Abstracts International: Section B: the Sciences and Engineering. Vol 55(8-B), Feb 1995, 3567, US: Univ Microfilms International.

87. Dishman RK. Compliance/adherence in health-related exercise. Health Psychol 1982; 1: 237–267.

88. Rippe JM, Ward A, Porcari JP, Freedson PS. Walking for health and fitness. JAMA 1988; 259: 2720–2724.

89. Goldberg L, Elliot DL. The effects of exercise on lipid metabolism in men and women. Sports Med 1987; 4: 307–321.

90. Blackburn H. Physical activity and hypertension. J Clin Hypertension 1986; 2: 154–162.

91. Dehn MM, Bruce RA. Longitudinal variations in maximal oxygen intake with age and activity. J Appl Physiol 1972; 33: 805–807.

92. Rippe JM, Maher PM, Ockene J. Care and rehabilitation of the patient following myocardial infarction. In: Rippe JM, Irwin RS, Alpert JS, eds. Intensive care medicine. Boston, MA: Little Brown, 1985: 366–376.

93. Porcari JP, Ward A, Morgan W. Effect of walking on state anxiety and blood pressure. Med Sci Sports Exerc 1988; 20: 85.

94. Laws A, Reaven GM. Physical activity, glucose, tolerance, and diabetes in older adults. Ann Behav Med 1991; 13: 125–132.

95. Kashiwa A, Rippe J. Fitness walking for women. New York: Putnam Publishing, 1987.

96. Dunn AL, Marcus BH, Kampert JB, Garcia ME, Kohl HW, Blair SN. Comparison of lifestyle and structured interventions to increase physical activity and cardiorespiratory fitness: a randomized trial. JAMA 1999; 281: 327–334.

97. Anderson RE, Wadden TA, Bartlett SJ, Zemel B, Verde TJ, Franckowiak BS. Effects of lifestyle activity vs. structured aerobic exercise in obese women: a randomized trial. JAMA 1999; 281: 335–340.

Chapter 3

Dietary Management of the Obese Patient

Sachiko St. Jeor, Judith M. Ashley,
and Jon P. Schrage

Diet therapy that educates overweight and obese patients about foods and eating habits is a key component in weight control. More than half the population in the United States is currently considered to be obese or overweight, making weight loss a major public health priority (1). It is not surprising that the prevalence of attempting to lose or to maintain weight is increasing in the United States (2). Obesity is also a worldwide concern that has been characterized as a "growing epidemic" with associated health problems and health care costs (3). Weight management and maintenance of overall health are both related to the quantity as well as the quality of what is eaten. Thus, the role of the diet in producing successful outcomes for the treatment and prevention of obesity is to:

1. provide essential nutrients to achieve and maintain an optimal nutrition status;

2. produce an energy deficit to yield a reasonable weight loss or to provide sufficient energy to prevent further weight gain; and

3. provide enjoyment of eating while supporting healthy eating patterns.

Dietary management is essential within an environment that promotes overeating, including a plethora of convenient, relatively inexpensive, highly palatable, energy-dense foods in large portion sizes (4).

Along with lifestyle changes of diet and activity, combined therapies include pharmacotherapy and surgical interventions as appropriate for treatment-resistant individuals (1,5). Treatment guidelines recommend a reasonable timescale of 6 months for a 10% reduction in body weight at a rate of 1–2 lb/week, 30 min or more of physical activity per day, and lifestyle therapy for at least 6 months before embarking on pharmacotherapy for overweight or obese adults, defined as a body mass index (BMI) ≥ 30, or $\geq 27 \, kg/m^2$ with two or more risk factors (1). However, it is important to note that more work is needed to demonstrate the long-term safety and efficacy of these weight loss medications. Surgical interventions also offer renewed interest for long-term outcomes for the severely obese, defined as BMI ≥ 40, or BMI ≥ 35 with coexisting morbidities.

Newer treatment recommendations now recognize obesity as a disease that is rarely, if ever, cured (5,6). There is a new emphasis on longer term weight management strategies and shorter term weight reduction efforts, accepting smaller initial weight losses of 5–10% of body weight as successful outcome goals (1,3,5,6). Further, long-term goals are targeted toward weight maintenance for the prevention of weight gain at any point and the assessment of BMI in normal weight individuals every 2 years (1).

Thus, the dietary management of obesity is one of the greatest challenges today, and newer strategies that will have longer term benefits are needed. Individualized behavioral approaches, designed to target major lifestyle changes in increasing physical activity and exercise as well as making healthier dietary choices, remain the hallmark of any treatment for obesity (7–9).

TRADITIONAL DIET DEFINITIONS

The major classification of diets for weight management has been based on the total level of energy (in kilocalories/day) provided. Dietary restriction represents the most conventional treatment, with diets defined as low calorie diets (LCDs) and very low calorie diets (VLCDs) as outlined below (1,3,4).

Low calorie diets usually average 1000–1500 kcal/day. The anticipated weight loss is approximately 0.5 kg/week or 1 lb/week for every 500-kcal/day deficit (4). However, the weight loss depends on the energy requirements of the individual patient. These diets focus on the use of regular foods, but usually incorporate formulated, fortified, and/or prepackaged and portioned products. Diets less than 1000 kcal/day often require vitamin and mineral supplementation (4). This approach has shown larger weight losses over time than the more severe energy restrictions (10). Reported weight losses on LCDs range from 0.5 to 1.5 kg/week (8.5 kg over 20 weeks) or approximately 2 lb/week (4), resulting in an average loss of 8–10% of body weight over a period of 3–12 months (1). Balanced deficit diets (BDDs) include LCDs that are generally above 1200 kcal/day for women and above 1500 kcal/day for most men (11). BDDs are considered nutritionally adequate because they can provide the essential nutrients by using a variety of well-chosen foods (4).

Very low calorie diets are considered to induce a modified fast, because they provide no more than 800 kcal/day (usually 400–500 kcal/day) (12). Regular foods are typically replaced with special formulated foods and/or drinks and supplements. Emphasis is placed on provision of 40–100 g (or 0.8–1.5 g/kg of ideal body weight) of protein of high biological value (HBV) to meet minimum protein requirements. Up to 100 g of carbohydrates, a minimum of fat including essential fatty acids, and recommended allowances of vitamins, minerals, and electrolytes are also needed. Although VLCDs can induce a more rapid weight loss, they can also produce more adverse metabolic effects and should be carried out under medical supervision. Reported weight loss averages 20 kg over 12 weeks or approximately 3 lb/week (4). Although initial weight loss is greater on VLCDs, studies of overall long-term weight loss (>1 year) show no difference from LCDs. Thus, LCDs and VLCDs have been found to be effective over the shorter term; however, weight regain generally occurs 3–5 years after treatment intervention ends (6,13).

DIETARY TREATMENT MODEL: SPECTRUM OF CARE

Medical advice and baseline nutrition assessment are always advised before embarking on any weight reduction regimen so that individualized intervention strategies can be developed. LCDs less than 1200 kcal/day should be used with caution because they may not provide the essential nutrients needed. However, at any point at which weight loss is desired, a BDD of greater than 1200 kcal/day may be initiated and is generally safe.

A treatment model adapted from the Blackburn Model (5) for obesity is summarized in Figure 3-1. The spectrum of care progresses in medical management as the severity of diet and combined therapies increase. This model emphasizes dietary involvement (assessment, management, and/or treatment as well as follow-up) at every stage. Even when used in the medical settings (primary care, medical, and/or surgical programs), LCDs and VLCDs may pose some unexpected burden on or consequence to the body, and a multidisciplinary treatment approach is recommended. Monitoring by a nutritionist (registered dietitian) is recommended at all stages, and physician monitoring and evaluation should accompany VLCDs and other restrictive or special dietary interventions. Dietary management is also important to the success of pharmacotherapy as well as pre- and postsurgical interventions.

The long-term basic approaches for prevention of weight gain or regain, in addition to shorter term approaches for weight reduction, include lifestyle management of diet and physical activity, which is essential and supportive to all. Current trends also promote the effectiveness of the primary care setting for earlier, less intensive interventions with support from the physician in conjunction with trained office staff (14,15).

It is well known that the majority of dieting individuals embark on weight reduction regimens without profes-

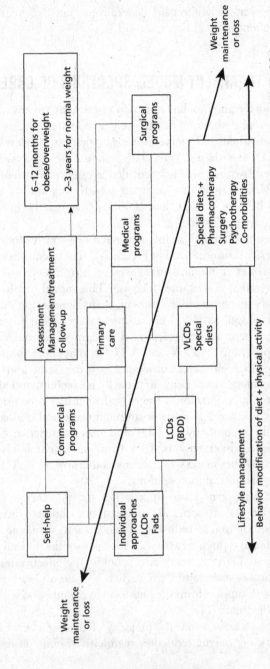

Figure 3-1 Spectrum of care for the treatment of obesity. (Adapted from the Blackburn Model from (5) p. 99.)

sional advice and will engage in self-help forms of treatment, including books and/or organized commercial groups. Generally, these are safe for individuals without medical complications over the short term and involve LCDs using a variety of individual approaches and diet fads that are in vogue.

In the new treatment paradigm, prevention of adult weight gain or regain is critically important. The saying that "if you can't lose, don't gain" applies to both the prevention of obesity in normal-weight individuals and exacerbation of the obese state in already obese or overweight individuals. Weight maintenance has been defined as less than ±5 lb over any two points in time (16). This concept of weight maintenance (or overall energy balance) should be applied for serious evaluation in 6-month intervals for already overweight or obese individuals and no less than 2-year intervals for normal weight individuals (1,3). It is also important to consider that weight maintainers tend to have healthier profiles overall (17) and that weight maintenance requires less intervention than weight loss and can concentrate on smaller, additive changes in behaviors, which may be more feasible to maintain.

NUTRIENT ADEQUACY AND BASIC 1200-KCAL BALANCED DEFICIT DIET

The focus of any diet is to provide adequate nutrition. The obese patient poses multiple and complex dietary challenges. The total energy (kilocalorie) intake is of central importance in weight management. Reductions in intake are too often accompanied by consequential compromises in essential nutrients and the overall quality of the diet. A major outcome of dietary treatment should be a qualitative improvement in diet, as evidenced by adherence to the Food Guide Pyramid the majority of the time (or at least 4 days of the week) (4). A basic 1200-kcal (4) diet adapted from the Food Guide Pyramid (18) can serve as an excellent starting point and is outlined in Table 3-1. The dietary pattern is based on the minimum number of servings recommended, with the addition of 1 teaspoon (4 g) of added sugar and

Table 3-1 Modification of the Food Guide Pyramid for a 1200-kcal Diet

Food Group	Number of Servings for a 1200-kcal Diet*,†
Bread group	6‡
Vegetable group	3
Fruit group	2
Milk group	2§
Meat group (ounces)	4¶

* Not recommended for pregnant or lactating women, children (depending on age), or those who have special dietary needs. At or below this low level of kilocalorie intake, it may not be possible to obtain recommended amounts of all nutrients from foods; therefore, it is important to make careful food choices, and the need for dietary supplements should be evaluated.
† This plan allows up to 1 teaspoon (4 g) of added sugar and 5 g of added fat.
‡ For maximum nutritional value, make whole-grain high-fiber choices.
§ Choose skim milk products. The discretionary 5 g of added fat can be used here to select low- or reduced-fat dairy products. With the increase in recommendations for calcium intake, if three servings from this group are encouraged, the 80–100 kcal additional to be provided should be accommodated.
¶ Select lean meat and use cooking methods that do not require added fat.
Source: US Department of Agriculture (18) and Committee to Develop Criteria for Evaluating the Outcomes of Approaches to Prevent and Treat Obesity (5).

5 g of added fat for flexibility, the meat group limited to 4 oz of lean, and use of non-fat (skim) milk products. Increased calcium recommendations emphasize the need for either an additional serving of the non-fat (skim) milk products (+80–100 kcal), which may need further accommodation or wise choices of calcium-rich and fortified foods. The adequacy of LCDs that are not carefully selected poses particular concern for intakes of calcium, folic acid, and vitamin B_{12}.

Calcium

The recent dietary reference intakes (DRIs) have outlined increased recommended levels for calcium which are higher than the 1989 recommended dietary allowances (RDAs) (19–21). The current adequate intakes (AIs) for both males and females are 1000 mg/day for ages 19–50 years and 1200 mg/day for ages 50 years and over (21). Practically speaking, it is difficult to achieve this level of calcium intake without consuming two to three servings of milk (approximately 250–300 mg per 8-oz serving) or dairy products (300–450 mg of calcium per 3 oz of cheese), dark green leafy vegetables (approximately 50–100 mg per half cup), nuts and seeds (25–75 mg per 1-oz serving), and calcium-fortified foods (200–300 mg per 8-oz serving, such as orange juice or soy milk) (22,23). All LCDs should especially encourage maximal intake of these foods, emphasizing low-fat lower calorie items. Related to increasing the bioavailability of calcium in the body is its dependence on vitamin D for absorption. It is important to consider the new AI level established for vitamin D, which increases with age (5, 10, and 15 μg/day for the two decades following 30, 50, and 70 years, respectively) as cholecalciferol (where 1 μg cholecalciferol = 40 IU vitamin D) (19,21). Thus, the level of vitamin D formerly recommended by the 1989 RDAs (10 μg/day to age 24 years and 5 μg/day thereafter) (20) has been significantly reversed with increasing needs for vitamin D recommended with increasing age. This stresses the need for adequate exposure to sunlight, which could be practically encouraged with recommendations to increase physical activity (such as walking) outdoors.

Folic Acid

The recent DRI (dietary reference intake) consisting of a new RDA of 400 μg/day of folate is more than double that recommended by the 1989 RDA (19,20,24). Dieting individuals are at particular risk for reduced intake of foods high in folate coming from "foliage", particularly fruits and vegetables. Thus, because of the evidence linking low folate intake with neural tube defects in the developing fetus, synthetic folic acid from fortified foods and/or supplements is recommended in addition to the food folate from a well-chosen varied diet in women of childbearing age (19).

AIs of naturally occurring folate in foods or synthetic folic acid supplementation in all adults is also viewed as particularly important in preventing hyperhomocystinemia associated with increased arteriosclerotic plaque formation and increased cardiovascular disease (24–27). Foods high in folate include leafy green vegetables, orange juice, and grain products (26). However, because of the inadequate intake of folate in general, the fortification of folic acid in cereals and grains starting in January 1998 was introduced as a significant public health strategy to help ensure better health for all Americans. Grain products were targeted for fortification with folic acid (140 µg per 100 g flour) because they are consumed by 90% of the target population. The effect of consuming six servings of folic-acid-enriched grain products has been calculated at 80% of the current RDA (four servings of bread = 160 µg, plus one serving of cereal = 100 µg, plus one serving of pasta = 60 µg, = total of 320/400 µg = 80% RDI) (26).

An upper tolerable limit of synthetic folic acid has been set at 1000 µg/day for adults aged 19 years and older to prevent masking of serious neurologic symptoms of vitamin B_{12} deficiency or pernicious anemia (24). The current level of folic acid in over-the-counter vitamin supplements is limited to 400 µg/tablet (28). Thus, it is important to target the five servings of fruits and vegetables as sources of folate in foods along with the six servings of folic-acid-enriched grain products to meet the current recommendations for folate. The upper tolerable level of intake still will not be exceeded with the consumption of 12 servings of fortified grain products, but vitamin supplements should then be used with caution. The new Dietary Reference Intakes (DRIs) that replace the old 1989 RDAs consider dietary folate equivalent (DFE) as 1 DFE = 1 µg of food folate = 0.6 µg of folic acid (from fortified food or supplement) consumed with food = 0.5 µg synthetic (supplemental) folic acid taken on an empty stomach (19,24). Thus, the best way to ensure adequate intakes of folate/folic acid DFEs, particularly when consuming LCDs, is by consuming a BDD meeting the minimum requirements of the Food Guide Pyramid as outlined in Table 3-1 and making sure the diet is rich in the best sources of folate-containing foods and folic-acid-fortified grain products.

Vitamin B$_{12}$

The new DRIs include RDAs for vitamin B$_{12}$ of 2.4 µg/day for both adult men and women over 14 years of age (19). These recommendations are higher than those suggested in 1989 (20). Because approximately 10–30% of older people may malabsorb vitamin B$_{12}$, current recommendations encourage persons 50 years or older to consume foods fortified with vitamin B$_{12}$ or take supplements (19,24). Clinical signs and symptoms of vitamin B$_{12}$ deficiency are not clearly exhibited in the elderly; many have undiagnosed deficiencies, and it has been recommended that suspected individuals not receive folic acid supplementation before their vitamin B$_{12}$ status is evaluated (29). Because vitamin B$_{12}$ is found in animal foods, consideration for protein adequacy is related, especially in older dieting Americans. Thus, LCDs should consist practically of no less than 50 g of protein, mainly from high biologically available and complete sources of essential amino acids, as provided by such foods as milk products, meat, poultry, fish, and eggs, which are all animal sources. Non-fat (skim) milk products are the best low-fat high-protein choices because of their quality of protein, high calcium content, and provision of other nutrients, including vitamin B$_{12}$.

DIETARY PRESCRIPTION: ENERGY BALANCE AND DEFICITS

When energy intake (food) equals energy expenditure [basal metabolic rate (BMR) + activity + thermogenesis], weight maintenance is achieved. Resting energy expenditure (REE) is currently measured in lieu of BMR using a variety of methods for indirect calorimetry. REE has been approximated to be 10% above BMR, accounting for 65–70% of total energy expenditure, or 24-h TEE (30). The thermic effect of food (TEF) and physical activity (PA) account for the remaining 10–15% and 20–30%, respectively, of 24-h

TEE. Because the 10% of kilocalories from thermogenesis (TEF), or metabolic response to food, is offset by the increase of 10% in REE above BMR, it is not figured into most formulas using REE.

The formula recommended for estimating total energy needs (24-h TEE) is as follows:

$$24\text{-h TEE} = REE \times \text{activity factor (AF)} + PA \text{ (24-h TEE)}$$
$$= REE \times AF + PA.$$

Resting energy expenditure can be calculated or measured by indirect calorimetry using a gas exchange system and special metabolic apparatus, such as the Metabolic Measurement Cart Horizons Systems (Sensor Medics, Anaheim, CA). Because indirect calorimetry is expensive and usually unavailable in general office settings, the following formula for calculating REE for healthy normal weight and obese adults (BMI 18–36) is recommended (Mifflin–St. Jeor equation, or MSJE) and is based on sex, height, weight, and age (30).

MSJE based on weight and height:

$$REE \text{ (men)} = 10 \times \text{weight (kg)} + 6.25 \times \text{height (cm)}$$
$$- 5 \times \text{age (years)} + 5,$$

$$REE \text{ (women)} = 10 \times \text{weight (kg)} + 6.25 \times \text{height (cm)}$$
$$- 5 \times \text{age (years)} - 161.$$

However, because BMI, or weight $(kg)/\text{height } (m)^2$ is currently being used in the assessment of overweight and obesity, work to convert REE to BMI units is underway. REE conversions to BMI by age and according to sex can be performed using the following equations derived from the same population as the MSJE for REE above (31). MSJE based on BMI:

$$REE \text{ (men)} = (BMI \times 28.15) - (\text{age} \times 6.41) + 1290,$$

$$REE \text{ (women)} = (BMI \times 28.15) - (\text{age} \times 6.44) + 905.$$

Interpretations of regression coefficients indicate the following influences on REE: a 28-kcal increase per BMI unit, a decrease of 6.5-kcal/year of age, and an increase of 385 kcal for men relative to women (31). Although work is in progress to establish an international REE registry to expand these charts, they can be usefully applied to project REE from BMI in healthy normal to overweight/obese (BMI 18–36) individuals aged 18–70 years and older, as was the population upon which these charts are based (32).

The AF consists of two components: a multiplication of the REE by an AF and an average estimated contribution of daily PA. We believe that the AF of 1.3 × REE projects the best estimate of energy expenditure for both men and women of sedentary activity, which includes most Americans (33,34). This activity factor of 1.3 × REE has also been recognized as the minimum value reflecting approximately 14 h of very light activity and 10 h at rest (20,35). Past recommendations have generally focused on recommendations of 1.5–1.6 × REE for light activity and 1.6–1.7 × REE for moderate activity, as set forth by the World Health Organization in 1985 (20,34), but these have been relatively high when used in our population (35). Thus, we have chosen to add an additional estimated amount of energy (kcal/day) contributed by a personalized assessment of physical activity, which is reflected by PA in the formula above. The PA can be calculated by those general activities and/or exercise patterns that can be estimated on a daily or weekly basis and approximates <4 to >7 kcal/min or 100–200 kcal/30 min, depending on the intensity of effort as outlined from Table 3-2 (35) and recommended for practical application by the most recent US Dietary Guidelines for Americans to encourage 30 min of moderate activity on most days (6).

For example, to expend 200 kcal, one must walk 2 miles at moderate intensity (3–4 mph), which should take about 20–30 min (35). Thus, the approximate amount of PA (kcal/24 h) expended can be added into the formula above either daily or averaged over the week and reflects a more personalized adjustment of the highly variable activity levels from day to day and from person to person. Two examples of these calculations follow. Note that PA can be figured either by the day or by the week. Intake can then be adjusted accordingly.

Example 1: A 50-year-old female office worker who walks 1 mile on her lunch hour every day of the week: height =

Table 3-2 Examples of Common Physical Activities for Healthy US Adults by Intensity of Effort Required in MET Scores and Kilocalories per Minute

Light (<3.0 METs or <4 kcal/min)	Moderate (3.0–8.0 METs or 4–7 kcal/min)	Hard/Vigorous (>6.0 METs or >7 kcal/min)
Walking, slowly (strolling) (1–2 mph)	Walking, briskly (3–4 mph)	Walking, briskly uphill or with a load
Cycling, stationary (<50 W)	Cycling for pleasure or transportation (≤10 mph)	Cycling, fast or racing (>10 mph)
Swimming, slow treading	Swimming, moderate effort	Swimming, fast treading or crawl
Conditioning exercise, light stretching	Conditioning exercise, general calisthenics	Conditioning exercise, stair ergometer, ski machine
–	Racket sports, table tennis	Racket sports, singles tennis, racketball
Golf, power cart	Golf, pulling cart or carrying clubs	–
Bowling		
Fishing, sitting	Fishing, standing/casting	Fishing in stream
Boating, power	Canoeing, leisurely (2.0–3.9 mph)	Canoeing, rapidly (≥4 mph)
Home care, carpet sweeping	Home care, general cleaning	Moving furniture
Mowing lawn, riding mower	Mowing lawn, power mower	Mowing lawn, hand mower
Home repair, carpentry	Home repair, painting	–

METs (work metabolic rate/resting metabolic rate) are multiples of the resting rate of oxygen consumption during physical activity. 1 MET represents the approximate rate of oxygen consumption of a seated adult at rest, or about 3.5 mL/min/kg. The equivalent energy cost of 1 MET in kilocalories/min is about 1.2 for a 70-kg person, or approximately 1 kcal/hr/kg.
From Pate et al (35) with permission.

64 inches; weight = 145 lb; BMI = 25. REE = 1258 × AF of 1.3 = 1635 kcal/day. Taking 1635 + PA of 100 (1-mile walk/day) = 1735 kcal/day.

Example 2: A 32-year-old male business executive who travels a lot, but works out two times a week for 1 h of vigorous activity (conditioning, exercise) at the health club and jogs two times a week for 1 h (5 miles): height = 70 inches; weight = 192 lb; BMI = 27. REE = 1828 × AF of 1.3 = 2376 kcal/day. Taking 2376 + PA of 120 (60 min × 2) = 120 × 7 kcal/min = 840 kcal/week = 120 kcal/day + 105 (10 miles at 100 kcal/mile) = 1000 kcal/week/7 = 143 kcal/day/7 2376 + PA of 120 + 143 = 2639 kcal/day.

Another way of monitoring daily physical activity is with an activity monitor, such as the Digi-Walker digital step counter or pedometer. The goal is to increase readouts in gradual steps by increasing physical activity. However, it is also important to document the type of activity being performed. The overall goal of such activity monitors is to provide a baseline reading and to motivate individuals to do more by providing them with direct feedback. Such increases in activity can then be more simply traced and recorded on self-assessment monitoring forms.

ESTIMATING DIETARY INTAKE AND PROMOTING CHANGE

One of the most difficult tasks in weight management is to estimate dietary intake. Most obese individuals underestimate their intake and fail to describe adequately their intake on a recall basis. Thus, at least a 7-day prospective food record is recommended for all potential patients to obtain as much detail as possible. This record should reflect the patients' "usual" or typical diet prior to intervention and should also document the pattern of eating (time, place, and occasion), portion size, and method of preparation. Patients should be instructed in detail about keeping a food record and counseled with regard to why it is important to establish a true baseline before any interventions. It is useful to tell patients that the value of the diet recommendation is directly dependent on the "honest" recording in the food records submitted for review.

The daily food record needs to reflect an accurate pattern on which to base any dietary interventions or recommendations for change (32). A general calculation for caloric intake can be done by categorizing foods into food groups, estimating portion sizes according to the Food Guide Pyramid, and separating out fats, sweets, and alcoholic and other caloric drinks for added caloric value. Special consideration needs to be given to mixed dishes that contain several food groups. The dietary intervention should begin with this usual pattern in mind. The first goal is either to achieve caloric balance to maintain weight or to achieve a caloric deficit to reflect a desired weight loss. An intervention plan can then be made using the Food Guide Pyramid, as outlined for the 1200-kcal BDD in Table 3-1 or by examples of the 1600-, 2200- and 2800-kcal diets outlined to guide healthy changes (17). Foods listed as eaten that are not listed conveniently in the Food Guide Pyramid are then targeted for evaluation jointly with the patient. It is important to be realistic about what can be achieved and what weight loss can be expected. Often patients have unrealistic expectations of their "ideal" weight. Thus, the usual food pattern derived from the food record can be used to begin a discussion about recommendations for change (increasing or decreasing food groups, assessing food portion sizes, changing or substituting foods especially of high caloric and/or high fat value, and changing eating patterns where feasible).

Our monthly monitoring chart is presented in Figure 3-2. This is an example of how self-monitoring can be helpful in reinforcing behavioral changes and encouraging adherence to prescribed dietary and activity changes. Patients are asked to fill out this abbreviated log daily or weekly including weights or weight changes and using a simple system of /, +, or—to indicate usual, more, or less than usual. In this way simple changes can be encouraged, monitored, and assessed. The goal is to encourage small incremental changes in behaviors toward the prescribed

Rate your meals in the spaces below (amount, servings) with "✓" or "+", or "–" for regular, more than usual, and less than usual.

	1	2	3	4	5	6	7	8	9	10	11	12	13	14	15	16	17	18	19	20	21	22	23	24	25	26	27	28	29	30	31
Meal tracking Breakfast																															
Lunch																															
Dinner																															
Snack(s)																															
Weight tracking +																															
–																															
Starting Weight ___ lbs																															
Fruits/vegetables # of servings per day																															
Water # of 8 oz glasses per day																															
PHYSICAL ACTIVITY																															
Behavioral changes 1																															
2																															

Ending Weight _____ lbs

Figure 3-2 Monitoring form for weight management program. (From Nutrition Education and Research Program, University of Nevada School of Medicine, Reno, NV 89557.)

BDD diet, with increases in PA monitored by a simple activity monitor (Digi-Walker) and awareness of weight changes. Patients are encouraged to record these weight changes using a scale at home, with the recommendation to weigh at the same time of day. This chart has been useful not only in our weight reduction programs but also in weight maintenance protocols.

DIET COMPOSITION

Although the ratios of fat, carbohydrate and protein continue to be the basis of most diet recommendations, the ideal macronutrient composition for weight loss and weight maintenance has not been established. Many new theories are emerging regarding the type and amount of fats in the diet, the role of carbohydrates beyond substitution for fat calories, the efficacy of high-protein diets for weight loss, the contributions of alcohol beyond its caloric load, the importance of water, and the impact of energy density on the selection of foods.

During weight reduction, it appears that the greatest impact of diet is from its total energy deficit, and the diet composition has little effect on the rate or magnitude of weight loss over the short term (36–38). On the other hand, it is important to note that over the long term or in conditions of weight maintenance, the total energy requirement may be affected by many factors and diet composition, mainly high fat intake, may make a contribution to weight gain (39).

While it appeared that a consensus was being established around the efficacy of diets low in fat, the increasing incidence of obesity despite lower fat intakes in the United States has raised many questions about the associated trends in higher total caloric intakes (40). Reducing dietary fat without reducing total calories does not result in weight loss. When food manufacturers reduce the fat in products, they often add sugars and carbohydrate to improve the flavor with little change in total calories. There is also a tendency to eat more servings of lower calorie foods than their regular calorie counterparts. In addition, many segments of the food industry have been increasing the portion size of convenience food and packaged products. The concomitant higher carbohydrate intakes are now also being questioned with regard to their relative efficacy compared to diets higher in monounsaturated fats and low in carbohydrates that have been demonstrating more favorable overall effects on risk factors, including high-density lipoprotein cholesterol, triglycerides, insulin, and glucose (41). Simultaneously, popularized high-protein diets continue to be suggested as an alternative, while the role of alcohol in weight management is largely ignored.

The effects of diet composition on total energy balance through increased intake and/or increases in energy expenditure through the thermic effect of food need further study and the role of fat intake on fat stores through selective oxidative processes and the genetic predisposition to gain weight and deposit fat centrally are important issues still to be addressed (42). Behavioral, psychological, and environmental factors also affect eating patterns and food intake, thus ultimately affecting diet composition. Additionally, physiologic stimulators as well as genetic factors may predispose the selection of foods higher in carbohydrates and/or fat. Thus, dietary patterns are highly individual and highly variable, resulting in unpredictable outcomes. Importantly, long-term compliance to dietary interventions is affected by how well the diet composition meets the most important of these established needs.

A low-calorie step I diet has been outlined by the recent guidelines for the treatment of obesity (1) and is recommended to guide the formulation of diets to be used for weight reduction while providing adequate nutrition. It incorporates guidelines outlined by other organizations and represents a balanced perspective that should be initiated in most cases (43,44). New additions are included for calories, protein, calcium, and fiber with the recommendation that alcohol be minimized because it displaces more nutritious foods. These guidelines are outlined in Table 3-3 (1) and should serve to guide the nutrient composition of LCDs used for weight reduction. They continue to be in accordance

Table 3-3 Low-Calorie Step 1 Diet

Nutrient	Recommended Intake
Calories*	Approximately 500 or 1000 kcal/day reduction from usual intake
Total Fat[†]	30% or less of total calories
Saturated Fatty Acids[‡]	8–10% of total calories
Monounsaturated Fatty Acids	Up to 15% of total calories
Polyunsaturated Fatty Acids	Up to 10% of total calories
Cholesterol[‡]	<300 mg/day
Protein[§]	Approximately 15% of total calories
Carbohydrate[¶]	55% or more of total calories
Sodium Chloride	No more than 100 mmol/day (approximately 2.4 g of sodium or approximately 6 g of sodium chloride)
Calcium**	1000–1500 mg
Fiber[¶]	20–30 g

* Alcohol provides unneeded calories and displaces more nutritious foods; it should be minimized.

[†] Fat-modified foods may provide a helpful strategy for lowering total fat intake but will only be effective if they are also low in calories and if there is no compensation of calories from carbohydrate or protein.

[¶] Patients with high blood cholesterol levels may need to use the step II diet to achieve further reductions in LDL cholesterol levels; in the step II diet, saturated fatty acids are reduced to less than 7% of total calories, and cholesterol levels to less than 200 mg/day. All of the other nutrients are the same as in step 1.

[§] Protein should be derived from plant sources and lean sources of animal protein.

[¶] Complex carbohydrates from different vegetables, fruits, and whole grains are good sources of vitamins, minerals, and fiber. A diet rich in soluble fiber, including oat bran, legumes, barley, and most fruits and vegetables may be effective in reducing risk factors. A high-fiber diet may also aid in weight management by promoting satiety at lower levels of calorie and fat intake. Some authorities recommend 20–30 g daily with 6 g from soluble fiber.

** Moderate weight loss may be associated with a loss of bone and thus may increase the risk of fracture. Many patients on weight loss diets consume less than the recommended amount of calcium and most mineral supplements do not supply adequate calcium supplementation, with 1000 mg calcium the rate of bone turnover during weight loss in premenopausal women. Dieters should maintain recommended calcium and vitamin D intakes during caloric restriction.

From Expert Panel on the Identification, Evaluation and Treatment of Overweight and Obesity in Adults, National Heart, Lung, and Blood Institute Education Initiative, National Institutes of Health (1) with permission.

with the most recent recommendations of the American Heart Association (AHA) for healthy weight, which recommend a match of intake of energy (calories) to overall energy needs with limited consumption of foods with a high caloric density and/or low nutritional quality, including those with a high content of sugars (45).

BEYOND DIET

Fat and sugar substitutes have a role in the dietary management of overweight and obese individuals primarily because they can potentially lower fat and caloric intake overall. However, it is important that they are used in the context of a regular diet, used in moderation and balance with other foods, are appreciated for total energy and nutrient value, and do not replace other nutritious foods (46,47).

Likewise, *meal replacements*, which are formulated products, have value because they provide a regulated amount of calories per serving, are usually fortified with essential nutrients and fiber, and are economical, safe, and convenient to use. They also provide a departure from normal eating patterns and can serve as a venue for re-education about and/or reformulation of what foods can be substituted or reintroduced.

Finally, *dietary supplements* should be considered when eating patterns are compromised, erratic, limited in choices, or less than 1200 kcal/day (4). Approximately 50% of the US population uses such supplements (48). The most common supplements are a multivitamin tablet, a calcium-containing supplement, and/or a vitamin C tablet. Vitamin and mineral supplements should never be used in lieu of a healthy diet, and their use should be evaluated on a case-by-case basis. Special attention should be placed on folate/folic acid, vitamin B_{12}, and calcium for dieting men as well as women.

Meal patterns and food portion sizes are also deemed important in regulating dietary intake overall and should be evaluated as part of the dietary history and 7-day food records. Interventions should be focused on the total diet, eating patterns rather than specific foods, and obtaining nutrient adequacy through a variety of foods. Finally, the enjoyment of eating should not be overlooked, and flexibility in a meal plan must be included to maximize the potential for long-term adherence rather than short-term compliance.

THE FUTURE OF DIETARY TREATMENT

While some patients will resort to pills and/or extreme eating behaviors, many will attempt to lose weight by following one of the many popular weight loss diets. Diet fads come and go, and there will always be a popular diet or dietary strategy that will appear to be monopolizing the marketplace. These fad diets may cause weight loss, but they may also pose a risk to a client's health. Education of patients toward realistic goals, maintenance of diet that comply with the dietary guidelines, and the rational that there is no one food, nutrient, or strategy that will be uniquely successful will always be a major challenge. The basic rule is that Energy In = Energy Out. For patients who want to lose weight, they have to eat less energy (less calories) and/or use more energy (physical activity).

Fad diets usually emphasize:

1. Large weight losses in short amounts of time.
2. Specific or "ideal" macronutrient composition of the diet (fat, carbohydrate, or protein).
3. Attributes of a special ingredient, food, or substance.
4. Rationale for a special mechanism of a food or food combination that is preferred.
5. Highly structured meal plans and recipes.
6. Foods or food combinations with special actions.
7. Focus on why other diets do not work.

Diet recommendations should be seriously evaluated with regard to efficacy, safety, and long-term effects. Although there can usually be some "half-truth" imbedded in any claim, the best way to evaluate a diet fad is by using the following questions (all of which should be answered "yes") (49).

- Is the diet well-balanced and does it include a variety of foods? Are all of the major food groups included?
- Does the diet impose a consistent caloric deficit or balance? Are the weight loss expectations reasonable? Is a safe weight loss (0.5–3 lb/week) promoted?
- Is a minimum of 50 g of protein provided daily?
- Is a minimum of 100 g of carbohydrate provided daily?
- Are the meal plans practical, flexible, and individualized? Does the plan allow for special foods and preferences?
- Is increased energy expenditure or appropriate physical activity emphasized?
- Are total kilocalories (energy) emphasized along with calorie sources of the diet (fat, carbohydrate, protein, alcohol) in an integrated lifestyle change approach?
- Are reasonable dietary goals established?
- Is nutrition education provided?
- Is positive behavior change for both diet and activity incorporated into the program?

It is important to recognize that the management of obesity is complex, with many underlying issues. There is no quick way to lose weight. Most of the weight loss industry flourishes without medical involvement. Approximately 62% of men and 71% of women are dieting at any one time, and these dieters include normal weight as well as underweight and obese individuals (50). An additional concern is that binge eating disorder (BED) occurs in 30% of obese people in treatment (51).

A long-term integrated lifestyle approach to weight control should include normal eating patterns and a variety of different foods. Obesity-related conditions, such as diabetes, hypertension, and cardiovascular diseases, should be carefully addressed and included in the dietary plan. Special efforts to maximize individual treatment are needed when the dietary management includes adjunctive therapies, such as pharmacotherapy or pre- or postsurgical interventions for weight loss. Caution should be taken to ensure adequate intake when patients lose weight more rapidly than anticipated with adjunctive therapies.

Importantly, losses of 5–10% of body weight are significant. Thus, interventions that encourage small incremental weight losses over time that can be maintained are proving to be more successful. A 200-kcal deficit per day (100 kcal in activity expenditure by 30 min of walking plus 100 kcal in intake by omitting 2 teaspoons of a high-fat food source) can result in 1400 kcal/week, equal to approximately 0.5 lb or approximately 26 lb over 1 year.

The dietary management of obesity is key to the treatment and management of obesity and prevention of further weight gain. The greatest challenge for health professionals is to develop innovative methods to help patients continue to enjoy eating while successfully controlling their weight. Further, as reimbursement for professional services are limited, patients need to assume responsibility in their own long-term care. Proactive consumer organizations, such as the American Obesity Association, provide education about obesity for the public and help professionals to provide the best possible care (52). They encourage insurance companies and third-party payers to provide adequate coverage for obesity treatment and prevention, especially in children.

The future of dietary treatment for obesity includes innovations to meet these new challenges. Because we have not been successful in the long-term, new treatment strategies must include the consideration of obesity as a disease. A seven-step process is recommended before initiating any dietary treatment for obesity.

1. Establish and assess BMI and related risks (waist measurements for men ≥40 inches and women ≥35 inches).

2. Assess weight-related comorbidities (diabetes, hypertension, cardiovascular diseases), readiness to diet, and any contraindications to a low-calorie diet (pregnancy, cancer cachexia, and other debilitating diseases).

3. Calculate and evaluate REE from BMI.
4. Estimate level of activity and usual activity.
5. Estimate dietary intake and/or establish a dietary intake pattern.
6. Project energy balance and prescribe a level of energy deficit and other dietary parameters.
7. Develop long-term practical dietary strategies and individual goals.

Thus, as the needs and future directions for the dietary management of the obese, as well as overweight individuals is better assessed, more successful outcomes will be achieved over the long-term. Short-lived unhealthy diet fads should be avoided, and emphasis should be placed on practical interventions that support health and the enjoyment of eating.

REFERENCES

1. Expert Panel on the Identification, Evaluation and Treatment of Overweight and Obesity in Adults, National Heart, Lung, and Blood Institute Education Initiative, National Institutes of Health. Clinical guidelines on the identification, evaluation and treatment of overweight and obesity in adults. Bethesda, MD: National Institutes of Health, 1998.
2. Serdula MK, Mokdad AH, Williamson DF, Galuska DA, et al. Prevalence of attempting weight loss and strategies for controlling weight. JAMA 1999; 282: 1353–1358.
3. World Health Organization. Obesity: preventing and managing the global epidemic. Report of a WHO consultation on obesity. Geneva: World Health Organization, 1998.
4. Hill JO, Peters JC. Environmental contributions to the obesity epidemic. Science 1998; 280: 1371–1373.
5. Committee to Develop Criteria for Evaluating the Outcomes of Approaches to Prevent and Treat Obesity. Food and Nutrition Board, Institute of Medicine. Thomas PR, ed. Weighing the options: criteria for evaluating weight-management programs. Washington, DC: National Academy Press, 1995.
6. Shape Up America and American Obesity Association. Guidance for the treatment of adult obesity. Bethesda, MD: Shape Up America, 1996.

7. Wadden TA. The treatment of obesity: an overview. In: Stunkard AJ, Wadden TA, eds. Obesity theory and therapy. New York: Raven Press, 1993: 197–217.

8. Foreyt JP, Goodrick GK. Impact of behavior therapy on weight loss. Am J Health Promotion 1994; 8: 466–468.

9. Stunkard AJ. Diet, exercise and behavior therapy: a cautionary tale. Obes Res 1996; 4: 293–294.

10. Frost G. A new method of energy prescription to improve weight loss. J Hum Nutr Dietetics 1991; 4: 369–373.

11. Eissenstat BE, Sigman-Grant M, Dolins KR. Weight management and cardiovascular disease. In: Kris-Etherton P, Burns JH, eds. Cardiovascular nutrition: strategies and tools for disease management and prevention. Chicago, IL: American Dietetic Association, 1998.

12. National Task Force on the Prevention and Treatment of Obesity, National Institutes of Health. Very low-calorie diets. JAMA 1993; 270: 967–974.

13. US Department of Agriculture and US Department of Health and Human Services. Dietary guidelines for Americans, 5th edn. Home and Garden Bulletin No. 232. Washington, DC: US Government Printing Office, 2000.

14. Wadden TA, Berkowitz RI, Vogt RA, et al. Lifestyle modification in the pharmacologic treatment of obesity: a pilot investigation of a potential primary care approach. Obes Res 1997; 5: 218–226.

15. Simkin-Silverman LR, Wing RR. Management of obesity in primary care. Obes Res 1997; 5: 603–612.

16. St. Jeor ST, Brunner RL, Harrington ME, et al. A classification system to evaluate weight maintainers, gainers, and losers. J Am Diet Assoc 1997; 97: 481–488.

17. St. Jeor ST, Brunner RL, Harrington ME, et al. Who are the maintainers? Obes Res 1995; 3: 249S–259S.

18. US Department of Agriculture. USDA's Food Guide Pyramid. Home and Garden Bulletin No. 252. Washington, DC: USDA Human Nutrition Information Service, 1992.

19. Yates AA, Schlicker SA, Suitor CW. Dietary reference intakes: the new basis for recommendations for calcium and related nutrients, B vitamins, and choline. J Am Diet Assoc 1998; 98: 699–706.

20. Institute of Medicine, Food and Nutrition Board. Recommended dietary allowances, 10th edn. Washington, DC: National Academy Press, 1989.

21. Institute of Medicine, Food and Nutrition Board. Dietary reference intakes for calcium, phosphorus, magnesium, vitamin D, and fluoride. Washington, DC: National Academy Press, 1997.

22. National Institutes of Health. Optimal calcium intake. NIH Consensus Statement 1994; 12: 1–31.

23. Mullins VA, Houtkooper L. Calcium supplement guidelines. Tucson, AZ: Cooperative Extension, University of Arizona, College of Agriculture, 1998.
24. Institute of Medicine, Food and Nutrition Board. Dietary reference intakes for thiamin, riboflavin, niacin, vitamin B_6, folate, vitamin 8–12, pantothenic acid, biotin, and choline. Washington, DC: National Academy Press, 1998.
25. Bailey LB. Evaluation of a new recommended dietary allowance for folate. J Am Diet Assoc 1992; 92: 463–468.
26. Hine J. What practitioners need to know about folic acid. J Am Diet Assoc 1996; 96: 451–452.
27. Rimm EB, Willett WC, Hu FB, et al. Folate and vitamin B_6 from diet and supplements in relation to risk of coronary heart disease among women. JAMA 1998; 279: 359–364.
28. US Department Health and Human Services, Part 3. Federal Register 1996; 61: 8750–8806.
29. Stabler SP, Lindenbaum J, Allen RH. Vitamin B_{12} deficiency in the elderly: current dilemmas. Am J Clin Nutr 1997; 66: 741–749.
30. Mifflin MD, St. Jeor ST, Hill LA, et al. A new predictive equation for resting energy expenditure in healthy individuals. Am J Clin Nutr 1990; 51: 241–247.
31. Harrington ME, St. Jeor ST, Silver-Stein U. Predicting resting energy expenditure from body mass index: practical applications and limitations [Abstract]. Obes Res 1997; 5: 17S.
32. St. Jeor ST, ed. Obesity assessment: tools, methods, interpretations. A reference case: the RENO Diet–Heart Study. New York: Chapman and Hall, 1997.
33. St. Jeor ST, Stumbo PJ. Energy needs and weight maintenance in controlled feeding studies. In: Dennis B, Ershow A, Obarzanek E, Clevidence B, eds. Well-controlled diet studies in humans: a practical guide to design and management. Chicago, IL: American Dietetic Association, 1998.
34. World Health Organization. Energy and protein requirements. Report of a Joint WHO/UNU expert consultation. Technical Report Series 724 Geneva: World Health Organization, 1985.
35. Pate RR, Pratt M, Blair SN, et al. Physical activity and public health: a recommendation from the Centers for Disease Control and Prevention and the American College of Sports Medicine. JAMA 1995; 273: 402–407.
36. Hill JO, Drougas H, Peters JC. Obesity treatment: can diet composition play a role? Ann Intern Med 1993; 119: 694–697.
37. Golay A, Allaz AF, Morel Y, et al. Similar weight loss with low- or high-carbohydrate diets. Am J Clin Nutr 1996; 63: 174–178.
38. Hill JO, Peters JC, Reed GW, et al. Nutrient balance in

humans: effects of diet composition. Am J Clin Nutr 1991; 54: 10–17.

39. Lichenstein A, Kennedy E, Bauer P, et al. Dietary fat consumption and health. Nutr Rev 1998; 56: S3–S28.

40. Connor WE, Connor SL. Should a low-fat, high-carbohydrate diet be recommended for everyone? N Engl J Med 1997; 337: 562–563.

41. Katan MB, Grundy SM, Willett W. Beyond low fat diets. N Engl J Med 1997; 337: 563–566.

42. Swinburn B, Ravussin E. Energy balance or fat balance? Am J Clin Nutr 1993; 57: 766S–771S.

43. National Cholesterol Education Program. Second report of the expert panel on detection, evaluation and treatment of high blood cholesterol in adults (Adult Treatment Panel II). Circulation 1994; 89: 1333.

44. National High Blood Pressure Education Program, NHLBI, NIH. The sixth report of the Joint National Committee on prevention, detection, evaluation and treatment of high blood pressure. NIH Publication No. 98–4080. Washington, DC: National Institutes of Health, 1997.

45. Nutrition Committee of the American Heart Association. AHA dietary guidelines revision 2000: a statement for healthcare professionals. Circulation 2000; 102: 2284–2299.

46. American Dietetic Association. Position of the American Dietetic Association: fat replacements. J Am Diet Assoc 1991; 91: 1285–1288.

47. American Dietetic Association. Position of the American Dietetic Association: use of nutritive and non-nutritive sweeteners. J Am Diet Assoc 1993; 93: 516–821.

48. Report of the Commission on Dietary Supplement Labels. Washington, DC: Department of Health and Human Services, 1997.

49. St. Jeor ST, Dwyer JT. The optimal diet: does it exist? Weight Control Digest 1991; 11 (7): 105.

50. Levy AS, Heaton AW. Weight control practices of US adults trying to lose weight. Ann Intern Med 1993; 119: 661–666.

51. American Psychiatric Association. Diagnostic and statistical manual of mental disorders, 4th edn. Washington, DC: American Psychiatric Association, 1994.

52. Atkinson RL. Let's give obesity the attention it deserves! AOA Rep 1996; 1: 1–2.

Chapter 4

Behavioral Strategies for Enhancing Weight Loss and Maintenance

Teresa K. King,
Elizabeth E. Lloyd-Richardson,
and Matthew M. Clark

The prevalence of obesity in the United States is increasing at an alarming rate, creating a major public health concern. In 1960, approximately one fourth of American adults were estimated to be overweight. At present, one third of American adults are estimated to be overweight (1). The factors that contribute to the prevalence of obesity in our society (a bountiful supply of inexpensive and highly appealing food, less reliance on manual labor at home and work, and sedentary leisure activities) seem to have established firm roots. Thus, the pattern of an increasing prevalence of obesity is expected to continue. This is extremely troubling given that excess body weight is a risk factor for coronary heart disease, the leading cause of death in the United States. Excess body weight is also associated with a host of other adverse health outcomes resulting in tremendous costs to our health care system (2).

BEHAVIORAL STRATEGIES FOR WEIGHT LOSS

Given that the societal factors contributing to overweight are not likely to change in the near future, nor have any miracle

pharmacological agents been identified, strategies are
needed which allow individuals to modify behaviors in a permanent fashion. Behavior therapy is the most widely used
formal treatment for losing weight (3). Behavior therapy is a
set of techniques derived from the principles of learning
theory. Learning theory posits that maladaptive behaviors
are learned through classical conditioning, instrumental conditioning, or modeling. Behavior can be understood in terms
of stimulus, response, and reinforcement. Whereas multiple
treatments for obesity exist, few of these have been critically
evaluated to determine their efficacy. Studies generally
support the use of behavioral approaches, whether alone
or in combination with a very low calorie diet or pharmacotherapy, as more effective than traditional approaches for
weight loss (2,4). The purpose of this chapter is to review
several key behavioral approaches to weight loss and maintenance. For each approach, we describe how the intervention was developed, i.e. we present the behavioral principles
which guided its conceptualization, we describe how
the strategy is utilized, and we review research on its
effectiveness.

STIMULUS CONTROL

Stimulus control is a term used to describe a set of procedures that seek to alter the antecedent stimuli that control
behavior (5). Stimulus control applied to weight management is directed towards modifying factors that serve as cues
for inappropriate eating (6). Initially, obese individuals were
presumed to be particularly responsive to various internal
and external triggers to eating, such as mood, time of day,
activity, and sight of particular foods (7,8). Further research
suggests that this increased responsivity to these cues is not
specific to the obese; targeting and altering an individual's
triggers for eating remains an integral component of most
behavioral weight loss programs for adults, as well as for
children (6,9–11).

Stimulus control strategies may be divided into several
categories: limiting the times and places associated with

eating, reducing exposure to food by storing it out of sight, limiting activities associated with eating, and reducing the purchase of problematic foods, thereby breaking "automatic" eating responses (9,12,13). In one study (14) participants were randomly assigned to one of the following intervention conditions: control group; standard behavior therapy plus experimenter-provided financial incentives for weight loss; standard behavior therapy plus experimenter-provided food; and standard behavior therapy plus food and incentives. Stimulus control strategies (specifically, eating in one place only, shopping from a list, storing food out of sight, and deciding ahead what to eat) were the only variables which predicted weight loss. Additionally, when combined with positive eating behaviors, such as making healthy food choices and limiting portion sizes, stimulus control strategies were the only factors that predicted weight loss and successful maintenance. By encouraging changes in these daily behaviors, new healthier behaviors may be learned and substituted for previously entrenched, unhealthy chains of eating behaviors.

SELF-MONITORING

Self-monitoring, defined as the systematic observation and recording of one's own specific target behaviors (15), is a critical component of any behavioral treatment for obesity (16,17). Through daily recording of dietary intake, and the circumstances under which eating occurs, information is obtained which allows the therapist to provide more accurate specific intervention strategies (9,18). Additionally, self-monitoring has not only been found useful in both assessment and treatment phases of weight management, but several studies have documented spontaneous reduction in caloric intake upon initiation of self-monitoring, presumably because of the increased awareness of food intake (12,19).

In a comprehensive investigation of the effectiveness of self-monitoring, Baker and Kirschenbaum (20) found monitoring food intake to be positively correlated with weight loss. Further, subjects who monitored more completely (e.g. all food consumed, time food eaten, quantity of food eaten, or grams of fat consumed) consistently lost the most weight. Lack of monitoring was negatively correlated with weight loss. These results are consistent with Sperduto et al's (21) finding that behavioral weight loss groups incorporating self-monitoring experienced greater weight reduction, as well as better attendance, than control groups not monitoring their eating and activity levels. Research confirms the need for consistent self-monitoring in behavioral weight reduction programs, not only to produce benefits such as increased awareness of eating behaviors and physical activity patterns and greater weight loss, but also to prevent failure in self-awareness and self-regulation (20,22). While there is no doubt that self-monitoring is an effective strategy, adherence can be a problem. Reminders to monitor may facilitate adherence. For example, phone calls and daily mailings encouraging monitoring assisted with minimizing weight gain during the holiday season (23). In addition, technological advances may facilitate adherence. Portable computer technology could increase the convenience of monitoring as well as provide prompts to remind individuals to record their intake. A recent study (24) used handheld computers to examine antecedents to binge episodes in obese women.

CONTINGENCY MANAGEMENT AND SELF-REWARD

Contingency management refers to treatment strategies which attempt to change behavior by modifying its consequences. Contingency management can be a useful and powerful tool in delineating specific target behaviors for change, as well as establishing criteria for success and consequences for both desirable and undesirable outcomes (25,26). Weight loss programs incorporating behavioral contracting have resulted in greater weight loss and lower attrition rates than programs not incorporating these elements (25,27). Inherent in the use of contingency management are the processes of self-monitoring, self-evaluation, and subsequent self-reward for goals obtained. Mahoney (17) investigated the contribution of self-reward, comparing treatment conditions of self-reward for weight loss, self-reward for habit improvement, self-monitoring without specific instruction in self-reward, and a delayed treatment control group. Results suggested that when self-reward, in the form of a refundable deposit, was added to the process of self-monitoring and self-evaluation, greater weight loss was obtained. Although results of this early study suggest that rewards targeting specific changes in eating habits, as opposed to rewards targeting actual weight loss, are more effective, this is not clearly supported by more recent research (28,29). Additionally, there is some evidence to suggest that subjects self-rewarding for achievement of goals are more likely to maintain their weight loss at 1-year follow-up than those receiving minimal contact or self-monitoring without reward (9,29).

Refundable deposit contracts are a common form of incentive used to facilitate behavior change, whether targeting weight loss, habit change, or group session attendance (25,30). Other types of incentives used include lottery drawings upon completion of group sessions and response cost procedures involving deduction of moneys for not achieving the specified goals of the contract. In their review of the literature, Brownell and Kramer (9) suggested that behavioral weight control programs incorporating incentives and self-reward, regardless of which type used, have average weight losses 30% greater than those programs not incorporating incentives. While there is great variation among the types of incentive programs and behaviors targeted in weight management, it is clear that use of contingency management and self-reward are effective strategies which should continue to be incorporated into behavioral weight management programs.

COGNITIVE RESTRUCTURING

Cognitive restructuring techniques focus on changing the errors in thinking which contribute to maladaptive behaviors (31). Behavioral treatment programs for obesity have incorporated strategies for changes in thought processes among participants (9,32,33). Not only does research suggest that cognitive factors may have a critical role in weight regulation (34), but alteration of these maladaptive cognitions may be related to control over eating, satiety, and dieting success (34). Based upon Mahoney and Mahoney's (35) early work describing maladaptive cognitions frequently experienced by dieters, common irrational beliefs are identified and modified in order to improve success at weight loss and long-term maintenance. Common irrational beliefs held by overweight individuals include: self-doubt over weight loss ("I've never been able to do it, why would I succeed now?"), establishment of unrealistic goals ("I'll never overeat again"); and punitive self-statements ("I'm a complete failure because I can't lose weight"). Individuals who hold more of these maladaptive cognitions and disparaging views of self are more likely to experience greater emotional distress and unhealthy eating patterns, which may contribute to difficulty losing weight and maintaining a weight loss (12,35,36).

Although cognitive distortions may be commonly experienced in obese individuals, research supporting the utility of specific cognitive restructuring techniques in weight management protocols has been mixed. Studies investigating use of self-instructional training (SIT), a form of cognitive restructuring involving identification of circumstances in which a dieter has poor control and then repeated rehearsal of appropriate self-statements, both imaginal and through practice situations (34), suggest no significant differences between SIT and "standard" behavioral treatments in either mean weight loss or alterations in cognitive patterns (24,27,37).

While research to date highlights the importance of cognitive factors on obesity and weight control, identification of specific clinically effective cognitive techniques is needed. Cepeda-Benito et al (38) have recently developed both state and trait measures of food craving, and while these have yet to be validated in an obese sample, they provide an example of a tool that may be helpful in assessing cognitive distortions and beliefs that could be intervened on within weight loss treatment. Incorporating appropriate cognitive outcome measures, rather than focusing on weight loss as a primary outcome, may shed light on the diverse cognitive processes involved in weight loss treatment and how best to manage maladaptive cognitions.

SOCIAL SUPPORT

Social support is often described as a critical component of weight management protocols (9,12,16,19) and is commonly included in one of three capacities (39): 1) teaching skills to participants in order to elicit and further enhance their social support networks (13); 2) actively involving significant family members in the weight loss process with the participant; and 3) eliciting social support as part of the group process. Nevertheless, the therapeutic effects of social support in weight management have yet to be investigated independently.

While involvement of significant family members has generally received mixed support, a meta-analysis of couples' weight loss programs (40) found couples' programs to be more effective overall than subject-alone programs. Peer and family social support have been positively correlated with successful weight loss and maintenance, although the mechanism involved in this relationship is unclear. However, Brownell et al (41) caution that simply having a cooperative spouse or family member does not guarantee improved weight loss. Brownell et al (41) found that subjects whose spouses participated in weight loss sessions and were trained in the specific techniques of modeling, self-monitoring, and reinforcement lost significantly more weight than either subjects with a cooperative spouse who did not attend sessions or subjects with a non-cooperative spouse who refused to participate in sessions. The effectiveness of social support may also depend on the gender of the individual trying to lose weight. Wing et al (42) found that women benefited more than men from a weight loss program which included spouses.

Explanations for the positive effects of social support include associations with decreased rates of depression and increased marital adjustment in couples participating together (40); increased instrumental support through the process of weight loss; and assistance with enhancement of self-acceptance and cognitive thought processes (27,43). Further research is needed on which types of social support are most helpful for successful weight loss. Retrospective investigations of partners of successful weight reducers, as well as those who are less successful, would provide information on which forms of social support are most effective, as well as what type of individual benefits most from inclusion of social support in a treatment package. Additionally, investigation of the role of social support, whether through extended family or community resources such as the church, may be particularly useful in improving successful weight loss and maintenance in minority populations (44,45).

WEIGHT MAINTENANCE STRATEGIES

It has been well documented that recidivism following weight loss is a serious problem (46,47). Some estimate that most patients regain all of their weight within 3–5 years (48). While numerous studies have documented high relapse rates for weight control, few investigations have examined innovative maintenance strategies. This section reviews the relevant research on behavioral strategies for weight maintenance.

Maintenance Groups

The foundation of current research into maintenance strategies was established by Perri et al in the 1980s in a series of studies (43,49,50). In these studies, the effects of professional contact, phone contact, relapse prevention training, social support, exercise and problem solving skills were examined. Perri et al (50) examined 26 men and 97 women who were 20–100% overweight and who participated in a 20-week group behavior therapy weight management program. During the 20-week program, participants were taught numerous behavioral strategies: self-monitoring, stimulus control, self-reinforcement, cognitive restructuring and slowing the rate of eating. After 20 weeks, subjects were randomly assigned to follow-up only or to four different 6 month biweekly maintenance programs.

1. A post-treatment contact condition which included weigh-ins, self-monitoring, and therapist-led problem solving of difficulties in maintaining habit changes in eating and exercise behavior. The problem solving training included four steps: problem identification, brainstorming, decision-making, and then solution implementation and verification.

2. A post-treatment contact and a social influence program. The social influence program included monetary group contingencies for adherence, participation in lectures, and instructions in peer telephone contact.

3. A post-treatment contact and an aerobic exercise program which combined a new set of exercise goals and therapist-led exercise sessions.

4. A post-treatment contact and a social influence and an aerobic exercise program.

Participation in these behavioral maintenance groups proved highly beneficial. At the 18-month follow-up, the subjects in the four post-treatment programs maintained 82.7% of their weight loss compared to an average sustained weight loss of only 33.3% for the subjects receiving follow-up only. Subjects in the combined maintenance condition maintained 99% of their weight loss, suggesting that the combination of high frequency exercise, coupled with support and problem solving, holds great promise in improving the long-term management of obesity.

Strategies Used by Successful Maintainers

One way of garnering information concerning effective strategies for maintaining weight loss is to actually examine individuals who have been successful at maintaining a significant weight loss and determine what behaviors these successful maintainers have in common. Researchers at the University of Pittsburgh School of Medicine (51,52) created a National Weight Control Registry (NWCR) of 629 women and 155 men who lost an average of 30 kg and had maintained a weight loss of at least 13.6 kg for 5 years. Fifty-five per cent of the sample used a formal weight loss program and 45% lost weight on their own. Most of the subjects (89%) modified both their dietary intake and their physical activity level to lose weight. The three most commonly used strategies to change diet were to limit the intake of certain foods, limit the quantities of food, and to count calories.

During their 5 years of maintenance, most subjects (92%) reported limiting their intake of certain foods. Many also reported relying on self-monitoring techniques by limiting quantities of foods (49%), restricting fat intake (38%), counting calories (36%) or counting fat grams (30%). Subjects also reported using stimulus control techniques. They ate most of their meals at home where food choices are more restricted. Subjects reported engaging in a high level of physical activity, averaging an equivalent of walking 28 miles/week. Subjects engaged in cycling, aerobics, walking, running and hiking. Thus, these maintainers participated in the type of physical activity which is recommended for weight loss, but the amount of time they reported exercising is more than double what is typically recommended. A recent telephone survey has confirmed this finding (53). Individuals who reported being successful with weight maintenance reported engaging in more strenuous activities compared to weight regainers. Interestingly, both groups reported similar levels of participation in mild and moderate activities.

Exercise

There is much support for the role of exercise in weight maintenance; thus, research has now focused on comparing the effectiveness of different types of exercise and on increasing the likelihood that exercise occurs. Researchers have found that instructing patients in home-based exercise rather than in group clinic-based exercise over a 12-month intervention facilitated weight maintenance at a 3-month follow-up (54). According to the authors, the greater convenience and flexibility of home-based exercise probably contributed to higher exercise adherence. During months 7–12, subjects in the home-based condition completed 78% of their exercise sessions compared to 48% in the group condition. Interestingly, subjects in the home-based conditions attended more weight loss group sessions and were more likely to complete food records. Thus, the authors speculate that exercise adherence may promote adherence to other strategies such as group attendance and self-monitoring of eating behavior, both of which facilitate maintenance. Extending this line of research, investigators have found that provision of home-based exercise equipment facilitates weight maintenance (55). Another recent study compared lifestyle activity (incorporating short bouts of moderate intensity activity into daily routine) to structured aerobic exercise in obese women and found no differences in weight maintenance (56). Thus, lifestyle activity may be a suitable alternative to aerobic exercise for maintaining a weight loss. The use of supervised exercise, personal trainers, and financial incentives have not improved long-term weight maintenance (57). In summary, convenience of exercise appears to increase adherence. However, research is needed to reconcile exactly how much exercise is needed for weight maintenance.

COGNITIVE RESTRUCTURING STRATEGIES

Cognitive restructuring strategies also appear important during the maintenance phase of weight loss. For example, it has been proposed that unrealistic weight loss expectations may contribute to relapse (58). If individuals are disappointed in their ability to reach their goal weight or discouraged with their rate of weight loss, these negative cognitions and emotions may reduce motivation and/or trigger overeating episodes. Recent research examining outcome expectations reveals the importance of challenging unrealistic outcome expectations (59). In a study of 60 obese women, subjects were asked prior to weight loss to identify their goal weight and four other weights: "dream weight" ("a weight you would choose if you could weigh whatever you wanted"); "happy weight" ("this weight is not as ideal as the first one; however, it is a weight that you would be happy to achieve"); "acceptable weight" ("a weight that you would not be particularly happy with, but one that you could accept, because it is less than your current weight"); and "disappointed weight" ("a weight that is less than your current weight, but one that you could not view as successful in any way; you would be disappointed if this were your final weight"). Subjects' goal weight averaged a 32% reduction in body weight. Despite a 16-kg weight loss during a 48-week treatment program, only 9% of subjects achieved a "happy weight". Furthermore, although they reported achieving numerous positive physical and psychological effects of weight loss, 47% still had not yet even reached their "disappointed" weight. Cognitive strategies to promote the adoption of a reasonable weight goal need to be identified by future research.

More evidence for the importance of cognitive strategies during the maintenance phase is provided by a study conducted by Kayman et al (60). These investigators found that maintainers incorporated a new eating style, but to avoid feelings of deprivation did not completely restrict their intake of problem foods. In contrast, regainers also dieted but did not permit themselves any of their favorite foods, and they viewed their weight loss foods as special foods, different from the foods their family would have and different from the foods they wanted. Thus, classifying foods as "good" and "bad" probably promoted dichotomous thinking and may have contributed to relapse.

Stress Management

Stress management continues to be important as individuals move from the weight loss phase to the weight maintenance phase of weight control. Kayman et al (60) found that regainers and maintainers reported experiencing stressful events at the same rate; however, the two groups differed in how they responded to stress. Maintainers used problem solving skills or confrontive ways of coping with stress. In contrast, relapsers used emotion-focused or escape-avoidance strategies such as eating, sleeping or just "hoping" the problem would go away. A basic component of most stress management interventions is training in problem solving skills where individuals are taught to identify problems, generate solutions, evaluate solutions, implement a solution and then evaluate the results. Thus, stress management strategies, in particular problem solving skills, may be important for weight maintenance.

Social support has also been identified as a weight loss facilitator (42). A support system can help one to problem solve, offer emotional support, or be available for practical assistance. Maintainers identify more support systems (61) and are more likely than regainers to seek support when dealing with stress (60). Recent research has explored new strategies to enhance social support. Wing and Jeffery (62) recruited overweight subjects, either alone, or with three friends or family members. The authors found that recruiting participants with a team of three friends and treating them with a social support intervention decreased dropout and improved maintenance.

In summary, continued contact with a professional, consistent exercise, social support, and maintaining dietary intake changes all facilitate weight maintenance. Behavioral strategies which have garnered support for their role in weight maintenance include self-monitoring (regular weighing, measuring and recording intake), stress management and problem solving, stimulus control, and cognitive restructuring. Whereas it is clear that there is a relationship between activity level and weight maintenance, it remains unclear how to foster the adoption of a more active lifestyle. Further research is warranted that examines the adoption and maintenance of an active lifestyle in an obese population. Preparing participants and practitioners for adopting a continuous care model of obesity should also be beneficial (Table 4-1).

CONCLUSIONS

Over 20 years ago Stunkard (63) summarized the literature on the behavioral treatment of obesity in the following manner:

Table 4-1 Maintenance Strategies

Physical activity
Low-fat diet
Coping skills
Extended treatment
Social support
Reasonable goal weight
Self-monitoring

Although behavior therapy has advanced the treatment of obesity, its results are still of limited clinical significance. Weight losses have been modest and the variability in results large and unexplained. Even long-term maintenance of weight loss which, it was originally hoped, would be a particular benefit of the behavioral approach, has not yet been established. One possibility of increasing the effectiveness of behavioral treatments is to combine them with other measures—dietary and pharmacologic.

Interestingly, the current status of behavioral treatments for obesity could be summarized in much the same manner. For example, in the vein of developing more effective treatments for weight loss, we have witnessed a rebirth of the pharmacologic treatment of obesity. Studies have documented the increased effectiveness of treatment programs which combine pharmacologic treatments with behavior therapy when compared to the use of the agent alone (2). A behaviorally focused treatment manual has already been adapted for use with the prescription drug Meridia® (64). Behavior therapy will undoubtedly continue to have an integral role in this movement.

While Stunkard's (63) quotation does still ring true, this is not to say the field has been devoid of innovation and progress. There have been some shifts in conceptualizing the treatment of obesity that will undoubtedly shape its future. The first is a shift from self-management to lifestyle modification. Behavioral treatments of obesity originally focused on self-control procedures, specifically self-monitoring and stimulus control (65). While self-control procedures are still an integral part of most weight management programs, the focus has begun to shift to a lifestyle modification approach that recognizes that in order to lose weight successfully the obese individual needs to establish a new lifestyle that supports the maintenance of a healthier and thinner physique (61,66).

Another shift involves goals for weight loss outcome or the evaluation of success. Behavior therapy has been described by Stunkard and other experts in the field as being of "limited clinical significance" because average weight losses are small. However, recent evidence suggests that losing even small amounts of weight (5–10% of body weight) can have a significant impact on health (67,68). The Institute of Medicine of the National Academy of Sciences (69) has defined successful long-term weight loss as a 5% reduction in body weight that is maintained for at least 1 year. Professionals are reaching consensus that losing 5–10% of body weight is a reasonable treatment outcome (27,70). So, rather than becoming disillusioned with behavior therapy because we have yet to develop a behavioral treatment that is effective at reducing obese individuals to "normal" weights, we have started to re-evaluate what it means to be successful. While behavior therapy can be evaluated as an effective treatment for achieving modest weight losses, patients may not view a 5% weight loss as a success (60). Thus, more research needs to be conducted so that patients can be convinced to accept smaller weight losses or so that treatments can be developed that produce larger weight losses which can be maintained.

There has also been a movement within the field of obesity treatment towards consideration of individual characteristics and recommending treatments based on those characteristics. Thus, rather than using a single approach with all obese individuals, there is an attempt to tailor or match treatments to individuals. For example, percentage overweight has been used to match individuals to treatment. Treatment recommendations are determined by their likely effectiveness and a risk–benefit analysis (70). Clark et al (71) found greater attrition from a low-intensity weight loss program among individuals with higher levels of obesity.

Factors besides level of obesity are also considered important when making treatment decisions. Schwartz and Brownell (72) surveyed experts in weight loss treatment to identify client characteristics important for treatment matching. Five factors were identified by a majority of the experts as important when making treatment decisions:

1. weight;
2. weight loss history;
3. medical condition;
4. eating disorders; and
5. psychiatric comorbidity.

Additional matching characteristics may include a history of sexual trauma (73) and a negative body image (74) as both of these factors have been shown to impact obesity treatment outcome. Intuitively, the idea of treatment matching makes sense; however, there has been very little empirical validation of treatment matching models. Research is needed that examines the validity and utility of treatment matching models for obesity.

A final shift involves the use of new technology to improve the delivery of weight loss treatments. For example, Internet behavior therapy programs have been designed for weight loss, which provide weekly information exchanges covering dietary, exercise and behavioral topics (75). While results are preliminary, Internet and email-based programs may be a viable option for treatment of mild to moderate obesity.

REFERENCES

1. Kuczmarski RJ, Flegal KM, Campbell SM, et al. Increasing prevalence of overweight among US Adults. JAMA 1994; 272: 205–211.
2. National Task Force on the Prevention and Treatment of Obesity. Long-term pharmacotherapy in the management of obesity. JAMA 1996; 276: 1907–1915.

3. Foreyt JP, Kondo AT. Advances in behavioral treatment of obesity. Prog Behav Modif 1984; 16: 231–256.
4. Wadden TA, Stunkard AJ, Liebschutz J. Three-year follow-up of the treatment of obesity by very-low-calorie diet, behavior therapy, and their combination. J Consult Clin Psychol 1988; 56: 925–928.
5. Mahoney M, Arnkoff DB. Self-management. In: Pomerlau OF, Brady JP, eds. Behavioral medicine: theory and practice. New York: Williams & Wilkins, 1979.
6. Foreyt JP, Cousins JH. Obesity. In: Mash E, Barkley R, eds. Treatment of childhood disorders. New York: Guilford Press, 1989.
7. Tuomisto T, Tuomisto MT, Heatherington M, Lappalainen R. Reasons for initiation and cessation of eating in obese men and women and the affective consequences of eating in everyday situations. Appetite 1998; 30: 211–222.
8. Ferster CB, Nurnberger JI, Levitt EE. The control of eating. J Mathetics 1962; 1: 87–109.
9. Brownell KD, Kramer FM. Behavioral management of obesity. Med Clin North Am 1989; 73: 185–201.
10. Haddock CK, Shadish WR, Klesges RC, Stein RJ. Treatments for childhood and adolescent obesity. Ann Behav Med 1994; 16: 235–244.
11. Wooley SC, Wooley OW, Dyrenforth SR. Theoretical, practical, and social issues in behavioral treatments of obesity. J Appl Behav Anal 1979; 12: 3–25.
12. Wadden TA, Bell ST. Obesity. In: Bellack AS, Hersen M, Kazdin AE, eds. International handbook of behavior modification and therapy, 2nd edn. New York: Plenum, 1990.
13. Wadden TA, Foster GD. Behavioral assessment and treatment of markedly obese patients. In: Wadden TA, VanItallie TB, eds. Treatment of the seriously obese patient. New York: Guilford, 1992.
14. French SA, Jeffery RW, Wing RR. Sex differences among participants in a weight-control program. Addict Behav 1994; 19: 147–158.
15. Kanfer FH. Self-monitoring: methodological limitations and clinical applications. J Consult Clin Psychol 1970; 35: 148–152.
16. Foreyt JP, Goodrick GK. Attributes of successful approaches to weight loss and control. Appl Prev Psychol 1994; 3: 209–15.
17. Mahoney M. Self-reward and self-monitoring techniques for weight control. Behav Ther 1974; 5: 48–57.
18. Wilson GT. Behavioral approaches to the treatment of obesity. In: Brownell KD, Fairburn CG, eds. Eating disorders and obesity: a comprehensive handbook. New York: Guilford, 1995.

19. Bellack AS, Rozensky R, Schwartz JS. A comparison of two forms of self-monitoring in a behavioral weight reduction program. Behav Ther 1974; 5: 523–530.

20. Baker RC, Kirschenbaum DS. Self-monitoring may be necessary for successful weight control. Behav Ther 1993; 24: 377–394.

21. Sperduto WA, Thompson HS, O'Brien RM. The effect of target behavior monitoring on weight loss and completion rate in a behavioral modification program for weight reduction. Addict Behav 1986; 11: 337–340.

22. Kirschenbaum DS. Elements of effective weight control programs: implications for exercise and sport psychology. J Appl Sport Psychol 1992; 4: 77–93.

23. Boutelle KN, Kirschenbaum DS, Baker RS, Mitchell ME. How can obese weight controllers minimize weight gain during the high risk holiday season? By self-monitoring very consistently. Health Psychol 1999; 18: 364–368.

24. Greeno CG, Wing RR, Shiffman S. Binge antecedents in obese women with and without binge eating disorder. J Consult Clin Psychol 2000; 68: 95–102.

25. Mavis BE, Stoffelmayr BE. Multidimensional evaluation of monetary incentive strategies for weight control. Psychol Rec 1994; 44: 239–252.

26. Stunkard AJ, Berthold HC. What is behavior therapy: a very short description of behavioral weight control. Am J Clin Nutr 1985; 41: 821–823.

27. Foreyt JP, Goodrick GK. Factors common to successful therapy for the obese patient. Med Sci Sports Exerc 1991; 23: 292–297.

28. Jeffery RW, Thompson PD, Wing RR. Effects on weight reduction of strong monetary contracts for caloric restriction or weight loss. Behav Ther 1978; 16: 363–369.

29. Kramer FM, Jeffery RW, Snell MK, et al. Maintenance of successful weight loss over 1 year: effects of financial contracts for weight maintenance or participation in skill training. Behav Ther 1986; 17: 295–301.

30. Sperduto WA, O'Brien RM. Effects of cash deposits on attendance and weight loss in a large-scale clinical program for obesity. Psychol Rep 1983; 52: 261–262.

31. Beck AT. Cognitive therapy and the emotional disorders, New York: International Universities Press, 1976.

32. DeLucia JL, Kalodner CR. An individualized cognitive intervention: does it increase the efficacy of behavioral interventions for obesity? Addict Behav 1990; 15: 473–479.

33. Bennett GA. An evaluation of self-instructional training in the treatment of obesity. Addict Behav 1986; 11: 125–134.

34. Bennett GA. Cognitive-behavioral treatments for obesity. J Psychosom Res 1988; 32: 661–665.

35. Mahoney MJ, Mahoney K. Permanent weight control: a total solution to the dieter's problem. New York: Norton, 1976.

36. Meichenbaum D, Cameron R. The clinical potential of modifying what clients say to themselves. Psychother Theory Res Pract 1974; 11: 103–117.

37. Yates BT. Cognitive vs. diet vs. exercise components in obesity bibliotherapy: effectiveness as a function of psychological benefits vs. psychological costs. South Psychol 1987; 3: 35–40.

38. Cepeda-Benito A, Gleaves DH, Williams TL, Erath SA. The development and validation of the state and trait food cravings questionnaires. Behav Ther 2000; 31: 151–173.

39. Parham ES. Enhancing social support in weight loss management groups. J Am Diet Assoc 1993; 93: 1152–1156.

40. Black DR, Glesser LJ, Kooyers KJ. A meta-analytic evaluation of couples weight loss programs. Health Psychol 1993; 9: 330–347.

41. Brownell KD, Heckerman CL, Westlake RJ, et al. The effect of couples training and partner co-operativeness in the behavioral treatment of obesity. Behav Ther 1978; 16: 323–333.

42. Wing RR, Marcus MD, Epstein LH, et al. A family-based approach to the treatment of obese type II diabetic patients. Diabetes Spectrum 1992; 5: 230.

43. Perri MG, McAdoo WG, McAllister DA, et al. Effects of peer support and therapist contact on long-term weight loss. J Consult Clin Psychol 1987; 55: 615–617.

44. Foreyt JP. Weight loss programs for minority populations. In: Brownell KD, Fairburn CG, eds. Eating disorders and obesity: a comprehensive handbook. New York: Guilford Press, 1995.

45. Klesges RC, DeBon M, Meyers A. Obesity in African American women: epidemiology, determinants, and treatment issues. In: Thompson JK, ed. Body image, eating disorders, and obesity: an integrative guide for assessment and treatment. Washington, DC: American Psychological Association, 1996.

46. Jeffery RW, Drewnoski A, Epstein LH, Stunkard AJ, Wilson GT, Wing RR, Hill DR. Long-term maintenance of weight loss: current status. Health Psychol 2000; 19: 5–16.

47. DePue JD, Clark MM, Ruggiero L, et al. Maintenance of weight loss: a needs assessment. Obes Res 1995; 3: 241–248.

48. Brownell KD, Jeffery RW. Improving long-term weight loss: pushing the limits of treatment. Behav Ther 1987; 18: 353–374.

49. Perri MG, McAdoo WG, Spevak PA, et al. Effect of a multicomponent maintenance program on long-term weight loss. J Consult Clin Psychol 1984; 52: 480–481.

50. Perri MG, McAllister DA, Gange JJ, et al. Effects of four maintenance programs on the long-term management of obesity. J Consult Clin Psychol 1988; 56: 529–534.
51. Klem ML, Wing RR, McGuire MT, et al. A descriptive study of individuals successful at long-term maintenance of substantial weight loss. Am J Clin Nutr 1997; 66: 239–246.
52. Klem ML, Wing RR, McGuire MT, Seagle HM, Hill JO. Psychological symptoms in individuals successful at long-term maintenance of weight loss. Health Psychol 1998; 17: 336–345.
53. McGuire MT, Wing RR, Klem ML, Hill JO. Behavioral strategies of individuals who have maintained long-term weight losses. Obes Res 1999; 7: 334–341.
54. Perri MG, Martin D, Leermakers EA, et al. Effects of group- versus home-based exercise in the treatment of obesity. J Consult Clin Psychol 1997; 65: 278–285.
55. Jakicic JM, Winters C, Lang W, Wing RR. Effects of intermittent exercise and use of home exercise equipment on adherence, weight loss, and fitness in overweight women. JAMA 1999; 282: 1554–1560.
56. Andersen RE, Wadden TA, Bartlett SJ, et al. Effects of lifestyle activity vs. structured aerobic exercise in obese women. JAMA 1999; 281: 335–340.
57. Jeffery RW, Wing RR, Thorson C, Burton LR. Use of personal trainers and financial incentives to increase exercise in a behavioral weight-loss program. J Consult Clin Psychol 1998; 66: 777–783.
58. Brownell KD, Wadden TA. Etiology and treatment of obesity: understanding a serious, prevalent, and refractory disorder. J Consult Clin Psychol 1992; 60: 505–517.
59. Foster GD, Wadden TA, Vogt RA, et al. What is a reasonable weight loss? Patients' expectations and evaluations of obesity treatment outcomes. J Consult Clin Psychol 1997; 65: 79–85.
60. Kayman S, Bruvold W, Stern JS. Maintenance and relapse after weight loss in women: behavioral aspects. Am J Clin Nutr 1990; 52: 800–807.
61. Head S, Brookhart A. Lifestyle modification and relapse prevention training during treatment for weight loss. Behav Ther 1997; 28: 307–321.
62. Wing RR, Jeffery RW. Benefits of recruiting participants with friends and increasing social support for weight loss and maintenance. J Consult Clin Psychol 1999; 67: 132–138.
63. Stunkard AJ. Behavioral treatment of obesity: the current status. Int J Obes 1978; 2: 237–248.
64. Brownell KD, Wadden TA. The LEARN Program for weight control, special medication edition for use with MERIDIA. Dallas, TX: American Health Publishing, 1998.

65. Stuart RB. Behavioral control of overeating. Behav Ther 1967; 5: 357–365.
66. Perri MG. Improving maintenance of weight loss following treatment by diet and lifestyle modification. In: Wadden TA, VanItallie TB, eds. Treatment of the seriously obese patient. New York: Guilford, 1992.
67. Blackburn GL. Effect of degree of weight loss on health benefits. Obes Res 1995; 3: 211S–216S.
68. Goldstein DJ. Beneficial effects of modest weight loss. Int J Obes 1991; 16: 397–416.
69. Institute of Medicine of the National Academy of Sciences. Weighing the options: criteria for evaluating weight management programs. Washington, DC: National Academy Press, 1995: 139.
70. Brownell KD, Wadden TA. The heterogeneity of obesity: fitting treatments to individuals. Behav Ther 1991; 22: 153–177.
71. Clark MM, Guise BJ, Niaura RS. Obesity level and attrition: support for patient-treatment matching in obesity treatment. Obes Res 1995; 3: 63–64.
72. Schwartz MB, Brownell KD. Matching individuals to weight loss treatments: a survey of obesity experts. J Consult Clin Psychol 1995; 63: 149–153.
73. King TK, Clark MM, Pera VP. History of sexual abuse and obesity treatment outcome. Addict Behav 1996; 21: 283–290.
74. Grilo CM. Treatment of obesity: an integrative model. In: Thompson JK, ed. Body image, eating disorders and obesity: an integrative guide for assessment and treatment. Washington, DC: American Psychological Association, 1996.
75. Tate DF, Wing RR, Winett RA. Using internet technology to deliver a behavioral weight loss program. JAMA 2001; 285: 1172–1177.

Chapter 5

Drug Treatment of Obesity

William W. Hardy and
Nikhil V. Dhurandhar

Over the past 10 years research has uncovered a myriad of
genes and gene products that have tremendous influence on
the metabolic processes governing weight. A better understanding of the physiology of energy conservation and
expenditure, appetite, satiety, the fat cell, regional fat deposition, and nutrient partitioning has opened doors that
should lead to new approaches to the treatment of obesity
(1–4). The importance of this research cannot be overstated.
There was a 50% increased incidence of obesity in the
United States between 1980 and 1994 and by the end of
1994, 22.5% of the population was obese [body mass index
(BMI) $\geq 30\,\text{kg/m}^2$] and 55% of the total population was
overweight (BMI $\geq 25\,\text{kg/m}^2$) (5,6).

The multitude of comorbid conditions that are caused
by or associated with obesity is daunting: type 2 diabetes,
cardiovascular disease (including atherosclerosis, fatty
myocardium with arrhythmias and sudden cardiac death)
(7–9), hypertension, gastrointestinal disturbances (fatty liver
which may progress to cirrhosis (10), hiatal and abdominal
wall hernias (11,12) and gall bladder disease), precipitation
or aggravation of arthropathy of weight-bearing joints,

central nervous system abnormalities (papilledema, increased intracranial pressure) (13), renal diseases which may progress to nephrosis (14,15), respiratory failure secondary to restrictive pulmonary disease (Pickwickian syndrome, right-sided heart failure), and/or aggravation of obstructive lung disease as well as sleep apnea, with its associated pathology. Soft-tissue infections, varicose veins, ulcerations, intertrigo and acanthosis nigricans are seen with increased frequency in the obese. Certain coaguolopathies, such as hyperfibrinogenemia, may be present with obesity (7). Postmenopausal breast cancer, gall bladder and genitourinary cancers and colon cancer are also more common (16,17).

Endocrinopathies associated with obesity include hypothyroidism, hyperadrenalism, polycystic ovary syndrome, hyperinsulinemia, hypogonadism, growth hormone deficiency, and pituitary dysfunction. Complications of surgery and pregnancy are increased with obesity (18,19). The psychosocial and work-related morbidity of this disease is incalculable (16,17).

Obesity is a serious illness. Despite the fact that our present approach has had limited success in coping with it, there is light at the end of the tunnel. The unraveling and better understanding through research of the multiple complex interreactive factors responsible for this disease may enable us to discern which factor or factors lead to a specific phenotype or an individual's presentation of obesity. This should allow more specifically directed therapy.

Physicians, in general, have been reluctant to prescribe medications for the treatment of this disease. A poor track record plus serious side-effects including the addictive or psychotic-inducing properties of the amphetamines, complications associated with some of the newer drugs (fenfluramine, dexfenfluramine) (20) and, most recently, phenylpropanolamine (PPA) (21) does not foster a great deal of confidence in drug treatment of a disease that many physicians still feel is solely related to a faulty lifestyle. For the most part, obesity has been treated with a calorie-restricted diet and "lose some weight and I'll see you next year". Encouraging increased physical activity, behavioral modification, and short-term drug therapy have been added by a number of physicians and treatment centers. These approaches have led to significant short-term weight loss in some patients, but long-term results have been poor. Regaining weight after a significant weight loss is well recognized but not well understood. During the 40,000–50,000 years' existence of modern man, famine has been a major factor in determining longevity, or the lack of it. It is not surprising that humans have developed many genetically determined traits to help them maintain body weight, resist weight loss during food deprivation and regain weight rapidly when food supplies are replenished. Increase in neuropeptide Y (NPY), the neuropeptide that elicits feeding response (22) and decreases in triiodothyronine and catacholamine activity leading to reduction in metabolic requirements in response to calorie restriction (23) are just a few examples of such responses. The multiple and redundant mechanisms that guard against weight loss probably interfere with the outcome of various weight management approaches by resisting weight loss or promoting weight gain in an individual.

Obesity management is further complicated by the fact that obesity is not a single disease but an expression of metabolic abnormalities generated by multiple factors. Overweight and obesity present in many guises. Fat deposition and lean body mass are variable. These variables are a reflection of underlying genetic and adaptive physiologic changes preceding and coinciding with the development of obesity. Sclafani (24) has classified the etiology of animal obesity into nine different groups: obesity of neural, endocrine, pharmacologic, nutritional, environmental, seasonal, genetic, idiopathic, or viral origin. At present, a reasonable or financially feasible way to determine the contribution of various etiologic factors in an obese individual is not available. As research continues, and the factors that are responsible for obesity in an individual are better characterized, we can anticipate more specific individualized approaches to obesity treatment (25).

Our current armamentarium for treating obesity is limited. Historically, the clinical treatment of obesity has been limited to a low-calorie low-fat high-fiber diet, an exercise regimen, and lifestyle behavior modification. It is estimated that many people who lose weight will regain most of the weight lost after 5 years. Although the lifestyle modification, diet, and exercise are most important for long-term weight maintenance and overall health, obese patients may need additional help. Admittedly, pharmacologic treatment of obesity is in its infancy, but research has developed some new and useful drugs that should help with the struggle to control weight. Before we discuss these, it is paramount to re-emphasize that the lifestyle change is the most important component in weight management. Without it, long-term success is highly unlikely.

In this review, we discuss the pharmacologic treatment of obesity, including a discussion of recently approved drugs, those still available, and others that may soon become available. It should be emphasized that in mainstream health care circles, antiobesity drugs should be regarded as supplements and not substitutes for the patient's effort at lifestyle change to improve diet choices and increase physical activity.

ROLE OF DRUGS IN WEIGHT MANAGEMENT

The goal of drug treatment is to achieve a period of negative energy balance followed by a balance of energy intake and output with minimal adverse effects. Patients frequently achieve the initial negative energy balance but it is too often followed by a period of positive energy balance. This is, among other things, secondary to the physiologic changes that take place with the initial weight loss and may lead to resistance of further weight loss. It has been documented that exercise may partially ameliorate some of this problem with greater sustained weight loss for 1 year in exercisers (26,27). Negative energy balance can be obtained by decreased energy intake or increased energy expenditure, or a combination of both. As the medications are discussed, the mechanisms of action are noted regarding the effect on food intake, alteration of metabolism or increased energy expenditure.

For the most part, obesity drugs used in the recent past are associated with weight loss for the first 6 months of treatment and then there is a plateau or resistance to further weight loss (28,29). There is a gradual weight regain if the drugs are withdrawn (28). Present medications have a relatively narrow therapeutic target compared to all the compensatory changes that the body can bring to bear in maintaining or increasing body weight when it is lost.

The ideal drug that effectively produces fat loss in an obese individual, prevents regain, and has no side-effects is not yet available. The response of an individual to currently available obesity drugs cannot be predicted. By profiling patients and evaluating their response to a specific drug, we may be better able to determine which type of drug would benefit which type of obese patient in the future.

MECHANISMS OF ACTION OF OBESITY DRUGS

Obesity drugs may act in one or more of the following ways.

1. Reduction in energy (food) intake.
2. Increase in energy expenditure.
3. Reduced absorption of ingested calories.
4. Shifting of nutrient partitioning from body fat mass to lean body mass.

A description follows of various mechanisms employed by different drugs used for weight management (Table 5-1).

Reduction of Energy Intake

Reduction of energy intake may occur in several ways. Most antiobesity drugs are thought to reduce appetite or hunger, so food-seeking behavior is reduced (30–32). However, increased satiety, resulting in reduced amounts of energy being consumed in a meal, or altered dietary preference is also possible. It has been shown that serotonin agonists may reduce cravings for carbohydrate (33) and dexfenfluramine may reduce preference for dietary fat (34). If the total

Table 5-1 Drugs that Reduce Energy Intake

Drug Group	FDA Approved	Duration	DEA Schedule	Trade Names	Dosage Form	Administration
CENTRALLY ACTING AGENTS						
Norepinephrine releasers						
Methamphetamine	Yes Warning box	Few weeks	II	Desoxyn	5, 10, 15	10 or 15mg. In a.m.
Amphetamine	Yes	Few weeks	II	Dexedrine	5, 10, 15	5mg b.i.d. to t.i.d.
Benzphetamine	Yes	Few weeks	III	Didrex	25–50	Initial dose: 25 mg q.d. Maximum dose: 25–50mg
Phendimetrazine	Yes	Few weeks	III	*Standard release:* Bontril PDM Plegine X-Trozine *Slow release:* Bontril Prelu-2 X-Trozine	35	35mg ac t.i.d.
Diethylpropion	Yes	Few weeks	IV	Tenuate Dospan	25, 75	25mg t.i.d. 75mg q.d.

Table 5-1 continues

Table 5-1 (Continued)

Drug Group	FDA Approved	Duration	DEA Schedule	Trade Names	Dosage Form	Administration
Norepinephrine reuptake inhibitors						
Phentermine	Yes	Few weeks	IV	*Standard release:*		
				Adipex-P	37.5	19–37.5mg q.d. in a.m.
				Fastin	30	15–30mg/day 2h pc breakfast
				Obenix	37.5	19–37.5mg/day 9 a.m.
				Oby-Cap	30	15–30mg/day 2h pc breakfast
				Oby-Trim	30	15–30mg/day 2h pc breakfast
				Zantryl		15–30mg/day 2h pc breakfast
				Slow release:	15, 30	
				Ionamin		15–30mg/day 2h pc breakfast (initial dose on left)
Phentermine	Yes	Few weeks	IV	*Standard release:*	37.5	19–37.5mg q.d. in a.m.
				Adipex-P	30	15–30mg/day 2h pc breakfast
				Fastin	37.5	19–37.5mg/day 9 a.m.
				Obenix	30	15–30mg/day 2h pc breakfast
				Oby-Cap	30	

Generic	Brand	Schedule	Duration	Controlled	Strength (mg)	Dose
	Oby-Trim				15, 30	15–30mg/day 2h pc breakfast
	Zantryl					15–30mg/day 2h pc breakfast (initial dose on left)
	Slow release: Ionamin					15mg/day ac breakfast (30mg for less responsive patients)
Mazindol	Sanorex	IV	Few weeks	Yes	1, 2	Initial dose: 1mg q.d. Maximum dose: 1mg t.i.d. w/meals
	Mazanor				1	Initial dose: 1mg q.d. Maximum dose: 1mg t.i.d. w/meals
*Serotonin–Norepinephrine Reuptake Inhibitor						
Sibutramine	Meridia Reductil	IV	Long term	Yes	5, 10, 15	Initial dose: 10mg/day Maximum dose: 20mg/day
PERIPHERALLY ACTING AGENTS						
Orlistat	Xenical		Long term	Yes	120mg	120mg t.i.d. w/meals

volume of food remains unchanged, reduction of the proportion of calories as fat will reduce energy intake.

Energy intake could also be reduced by reduction of absorption of nutrients from the gastrointestinal tract, in effect producing malabsorption, as described below.

Increase in Energy Expenditure

Obesity drugs may increase energy expenditure by stimulating an increase in activity levels or by increasing metabolic rate directly. Some patients complain of tremor, particularly during the initial phase of treatment with certain pharmacologic agents (35,36). Tremor is muscle contraction and requires energy expenditure. Anecdotally, patients report an increase in willingness to exercise and feel more comfortable when active, but this has not been clearly documented. Most studies include behavioral therapy that focuses on increasing activity, so the independent contribution of medications is difficult to determine.

Animal and human studies suggest that some obesity drugs may increase energy expenditure by increasing resting metabolic rate (RMR), whereas others report increased dietary-induced thermogenesis (DIT) (31,37–39). The combination of ephedrine and caffeine has been shown to increase energy expenditure, possibly by stimulating β-adrenergic receptors (37,38). Compared to the untreated control group, rats given fenfluramine had a normal RMR but an exaggerated rise in energy expenditure in response to a meal (31). Troiano et al (39) demonstrated a similar phenomenon in humans. However, other investigators have found no increase in either RMR or in DIT with fenfluramine or dexfenfluramine (40).

Decreased Absorption

Interfering with digestion and/or absorption of macronutrients results in reduced availability of calories from the ingested food. A drug could inhibit a digestive enzyme or bind to its substrate (nutrient) and inhibit digestion and/or absorption. Drugs that reduce the digestion of dietary carbohydrates and fats by inhibiting the digestive enzymes are available and are discussed below. Chitosan is postulated to reduce dietary fat absorption by binding with the fat. Most of the side-effects of the drugs reducing digestion or absorption are caused by the increased amounts of undigested nutrients reaching the large intestines. Drugs currently available in this category do not act centrally and therefore may be safer.

Nutrient Partitioning

It is considered that reducing the amount of *de novo* fat synthesis from macronutrients would reduce body fat stores. Hydroxycitric acid, an ingredient in the fruit *Garcinia cambogia* is a potent inhibitor of citrate lyase. Citrate lyase is a key enzyme in *de novo* lipogenesis and inhibition of this enzyme is postulated to result in reduced fat mass and body weight. Results of the clinical trials with hydroxycitric acid for weight loss are discussed below.

CATEGORIES OF OBESITY DRUGS

Centrally Acting Obesity Drugs

Adrenergic Stimulation α-I, -II, β-I, -II, and -III adrenoreceptors all have an effect on food intake, satiety and/or metabolism. Inhibition of food intake can be achieved by agonists of α-I or β-II adrenergic receptors.

Amphetamine and methamphetamine are Drug Enforcement Agency (DEA) Schedule II drugs which are rarely used because of their abuse potential and the reported psychotic reactions. They are no more effective than potentially less abusive drugs of the same class. All the amphetamine-like drugs are stimulants, which may lead to problems with blood pressure, tremor, dry mouth, constipation, and insomnia. These drugs have an anorectic effect by modulating the noradrenergic neurotransmission and a probable addictive effect through dopaminergic transmission.

Benzphetamine, phendimetrazine, chlorphentermine, and chlortermine are Schedule III drugs that have less abuse potential but are not very popular with practicing physicians. Adrenergics in the DEA Class IV include medications frequently used on a short-term basis in the United States. These include phentermine, diethylpropion and mazindol. Phentermine and diethylpropion stimulate release of norepinephrine from nerve terminals in the central nervous system. Mazindol inhibits reuptake of norepinephrine. All three of these drugs have minimal addiction or abuse potential (41). Griffiths et al (41) demonstrated in non-human primates that diethylpropion had somewhat higher reinforcement potential than did phentermine. Silverstone (32) concluded that all of the drugs in this category produce approximately the same weight loss.

Some over-the-counter obesity drugs contain PPA which has α-catacholamine agonist action in the parventricular nucleus causing a decrease in food intake. PPA, found in appetite suppressants and in cough and cold medications, has been shown to be an independent risk factor for hemorrhagic stroke (21) and recently preparations containing PPA have been withdrawn from the market by the Food and Drug Administration (FDA) (http://www.fda.gov/cder/drug/infopage/ppa/default.htm).

Serotonergic Stimulation Sibutramine is the only currently approved obesity drug that prevents the reuptake of serotonin in the neural clefts. Fluoxetine and sertraline are specific serotonin reuptake inhibitors not approved specifically by the FDA for weight loss or appetite control but that have been demonstrated to reduce food intake in animals and have been shown to produce weight loss in humans in short-term trials. However, weight returned to pretreatment levels after 1 year (42). Recently the FDA approved the use of fluoxetine in the eating disorder bulimia nervosa (http://vm.cfsan.fda.gov/dms/fdeatdis.html).

Adrenergic and Serotonergic Stimulation The combination of fenfluramine, a serotonin agonist, and phentermine, an adrenergic agonist, was first reported in 1984 by Weintraub et al (43). Fenfluramine or dexfenfluramine in combination with phentermine (fen–phen) enjoyed short-term success in the treatment of obesity (28,29,44). The combination is no longer available as dexfenfluramine and fenfluramine have been taken off the market because of the development of left heart valvulopathy in a significant number of patients taking these drugs (20). Other side-effects associated with the fenfluramine component of this combination included possible pulmonary hypertension, short-term memory loss, and the serotonin syndrome. Fenfluramine and its major metabolite (D-norphenfluramine) released serotonin from nerve endings and also blocked its reuptake. The combination of fen–phen was highly effective in producing weight loss and its absence from our armamentarium has left quite a vacuum.

Many practicing physicians have used fluoxetine or other selective serotonin reuptake inhibitors, which have excellent side-effect profiles, in combination with phentermine (45) in an attempt to duplicate the results of fen–phen (29).

Sibutramine was initially evaluated as an antidepressant because of its ability to inhibit the reuptake of norepinephrine and serotonin in a manner similar to other antidepressants such as venlafaxine. Sibutramine was found to be associated with weight loss and was not that effective as an antidepressant. The drug is now marketed for weight loss. It has the advantage of a combination of adrenergic- and serotonergic-like activity. Sibutramine inhibits serotonin reuptake in a manner similar to that of the selective serotonin reuptake inhibitors. Unlike fenfluramine, it does not cause release of serotonin. Sibutramine has no dopaminergic effects, and no evidence of addictive potential. Sibutramine is associated with decreased appetite and increased satiety (46). Animal studies have demonstrated increases in metabolic rate for more than 6 h after the drug was given. Side-effects associated with noradrenergic agonists include insomnia, nervousness, dry mouth, and constipation. They can also affect blood pressure, cause increased heart rate, and palpitations. A history of coronary disease, congestive heart failure and/or arrhythmias as well as stroke or transient ischemic attack would preclude the use of this medication. Serotonergic drugs are not indicated for use with other selective serotonin reuptake inhibitors which may precipitate the serotonin syndrome (47), or with monoamine oxidase inhibitors.

Peripherally Acting Agents

Orlistat is a pancreatic lipase-binding agent that reduces fat absorption in the gastrointestinal tract (48,49). The drug, recently approved by United States FDA, is essentially not absorbed systemically, and its side-effects are limited to those resulting from the inhibition of dietary fat absorption. Increased gas and flatulence, cramping, diarrhea, oily rectal discharge and soilage are common, particularly in the initial period of treatment. These side-effects improve with time and reductions of the indiscretions in the diet which may precede them. About one third of the dietary fat absorption is blocked by orlistat with concomitant caloric loss in the stool. In a diet containing 30% calories as fat, this can lead to a significant relative negative energy balance. Fat-soluble vitamin supplements are recommended with the use of orlistat with an appropriate interval between the vitamin and lipase inhibitor intake.

Experimental and/or Drugs Not Currently Approved for Obesity Treatment

Acarbose is an α-glucosidase inhibitor that reduces digestion of complex carbohydrates leading to undigested food stuffs entering the colon (50). This is associated with cramping, gas, abdominal discomfort, and diarrhea. This drug is approved for the treatment of diabetes in the United States but has not been very effective in weight loss trials.

Chitosan is a product promoted through the health food industry. This is a polymer of glucosamine extracted from mollusk shells and reportedly reduces fat absorption by binding dietary fat. Studies in animals on high-fat diets revealed chitosan prevented weight gain, fatty liver, and hyperlipidemia. Studies in humans are limited and not very impressive (51).

Ephedrine, a centrally and peripherally acting non-specific β-adrenergic stimulator, has been used alone and in combination with caffeine and/or aspirin in the treatment of obesity. Ephedrine directly stimulates β-adrenergic receptors and also stimulates the sympathetic nerve terminal release of norepinephrine. Caffeine delays the degradation of ephedrine and inhibits the postsynaptic phosphodiesterase, thereby potentiating the effect of ephedrine. Caffeine also causes a mild increase in thermogenesis. Aspirin potentiates and prolongs the norepinephrine activity by interfering with prostaglandins, which degrade norepinephrine in the neural cleft. The non-specific nature of the β-agonist stimulation effect on β-I and -II receptors may cause an increased blood pressure and/or heart rate as well as nervousness and tremor during the initial phase of treatment. There is also an associated rise in serum insulin levels. Tachyphylaxis usually eliminates the symptoms related to the β-I and -II stimulation within 1 month, but there is evidence that the β-III stimulation continues, as the increase in metabolic rate persists. There are many studies confirming these findings (37,38,52).

There is currently concern regarding the health food industry's marketing of supplements that contain these three ingredients: Ma Huang, a Chinese herb containing ephedrine; coffee beans; and acetosalicylic acid from willow bark. Because such extracts may be marketed as "supplements" in the United States and are subject to minimal FDA oversight, sales of varieties of this combination are currently booming. The FDA and Federal Trade Commission (FTC) have become concerned and issued warnings because a number of people have had cardiac events or even died while taking these compounds (53), but a direct cause and effect relationship has not been established.

Conjugated linoleic acid has been shown to increase lean body mass in animals, especially in growing young animals. Trials of this medication on weight loss have not been effective; however, there are ongoing trials to determine if a regain in weight would be more likely to be lean body mass rather than adipose tissue (54,55).

Green tea extract contains caffeine and catechin polyphenols, which have been found to increase peripheral thermogenesis. A small study in humans revealed a 3.4% increase in 24-h energy expenditure, and a 25% increase in the fat oxidation (56). Studies on weight loss have not been reported.

Hydroxycitric acid plays a part in inhibiting *de novo* lipogenesis. Hydroxycitric acid is the active ingredient of the fruit *Garcinia cambogia*. Therefore, hydroxy citrate and *Garcinia cambogia* are hypothesized to have a role in weight loss. However, a 12-week randomized double-blind placebo-controlled trial in 135 overweight men and women failed to show significant weight loss differences that could be attributed to *Garcinia cambogia* (57).

Potassium, magnesium, and phosphate in orange juice reportedly increase the thermic effect of food in overweight women (58,59). Obesity has been associated with decreased levels of skeletal muscle potassium and serum phosphate. The authors of these studies (58,59) assumed that the pool of potassium, magnesium, and phosphate is low in obesity and replenishing these minerals may increase thermogenesis. Potassium, magnesium, and phosphate electrolytes were added to orange juice. This combination facilitates the intercellular transfer of potassium with the insulin and increases the sodium/potassium adenosine triphosphatase activity, which has high energy cost. A 6.3% increase in energy expenditure was noted in 30 min in the electrolyte plus orange juice group compared to the group receiving only orange juice. Further studies of this phenomenon may be in order.

Metformin, a biguanide oral antihyperglycemic drug is known to improve insulin sensitivity as well as decrease static glucose production and decrease intestinal glucose absorption. Obesity is known to be associated with hyperinsulinemia and insulin resistance. Studies indicate that it may be useful in inhibiting food intake, lowering body weight and body fat in the non-diabetic obese patient as well as the diabetic (60–62). It has been effective in some of the metabolic abnormalities associated with polycystic ovary syndrome.

Topiramate is an antiepileptic drug which has recently become available in the United States and in many European countries and it is indicated in partial-onset seizures. It was noted that "weight loss" and "anorexia" were two of the side-effects of the drug, along with central nervous system related symptoms such as dizziness, fatigue, visual disturbances, ataxia, impaired concentration, and nephrolithiasis (63,64). The effect of topiramate on body weight has received significant attention. Many antiepileptic drugs are known to increase body weight and the observation of topiramate-induced weight loss may have application in weight reduction of some obese patients, particularly in treating patients with mood disorders and obesity as well as some binge eaters (65,66).

Cytomel: triiodothyronine (T3) levels have been noted to decrease with rapid weight loss, starvation or restricted caloric intake. There is a concomitant increase in reverse T3 which is much less metabolically active. Attempts to treat this drop in T3 with cytomel has led to slight increases in weight loss but also to increased muscle catabolism, the additional weight loss being at the expense of lean body mass and not adipose tissue (67,68). Cytomel is not recommended at this time, but further studies may be in order. Previous history of thyroid hormone (T4) treatment for obesity was met with less than satisfactory results and significant side-effects, and is no longer considered an option.

Leptin, the hormone secreted by adipocytes, was discovered in 1994 and acts directly or indirectly through specific receptors in the central nervous system to decrease food intake and increase energy expenditure. It also influences glucose and fat metabolism and has other neuroendocrine functions. The multiple targets of leptin and its interactions in the central nervous system and periphery have opened a vast number of pathways that affect energy balance (25,69). The optimism about the role of leptin in the treatment of human obesity was dampened by the findings that most obese humans have elevated levels of leptin (70). However, a recently published clinical trial of leptin injections vs. placebo showed a significant dose–response effect for weight loss in the leptin group (71). Weight loss produced in 24 weeks in the highest dose leptin group was 7.1 kg, compared to 1.7 kg in the placebo group.

CRITERIA FOR RECEIVING OBESITY DRUGS

In 1996 the National Institutes of Health Taskforce on the Prevention and Treatment of Obesity did not recommend long-term drug therapy for obesity until additional research had been performed (72). The FDA guidelines stipulated a BMI of $30 \, kg/m^2$ ($27 \, kg/m^2$ with comorbidities) or more be used as a basis for considering drug therapy (73). In 1995, the North American Association for the Study of Obesity (NAASO) convened a board including members from the FDA and National Institutes of Health (NIH) suggesting a slightly lower limit of BMI (74). However, more recently, NAASO endorsed the National Heart, Lung, and Blood Institute (NHLBI) guidelines (75), which set the BMI thresholds for treatment somewhat higher. Shape Up America! and the American Obesity Association have added their recommendations (76). According to the NHLBI guidelines, which are the most recent guidelines, individuals with a BMI of 25–29.9 are considered overweight, and individuals with a BMI $\geq$ 30 are considered obese. Treatment of overweight with drugs is recommended only when two or more risk factors are present. An initial goal for weight loss might be 10% weight loss below baseline and, upon reaching the goal, further weight loss may be attempted if indicated by further evaluation. The rate of weight loss should be about 0.5–1 kg/week. Greater rates of weight loss may compromise safety. The guidelines further state that weight loss and maintenance therapy should use the combination of reduced calories, increased physical activity, and behavior therapy. As an adjunct to this strategy, weight loss drugs approved by the FDA may be used for patients with a BMI $\geq$ 30 with no concomitant obesity-related risk factors or for patients with a BMI $\geq$ 27 with concomitant obesity-related risk factors. The lifestyle changes which are essential for long-term success must be a priority. Physicians must pay close attention to appropriately screening candidates suitable for drug treatment of obesity and should also be very vigilant about noting adverse effects, if any, of the pharmacotherapy. The relative and absolute contraindications to drug therapy are listed (Table 5-2).

CRITERIA FOR SUCCESSFUL WEIGHT LOSS

Weight loss is a surrogate measure used to define fat loss. Present evidence points to fat loss as the measurement

Table 5-2 Contraindications or Cautions to the Use of Obesity Drugs

1. Pregnancy or lactation
2. Unstable cardiac disease
3. Uncontrolled hypertension
4. Unstable severe systemic illness
5. Unstable psychiatric disorder or anorexia
6. Other drug therapy, if incompatible (e.g. monoamine oxidase inhibitors, migraine drugs)
7. Closed angle glaucoma (caution)
8. General anesthesia (absolute contraindication, except emergencies)

related to beneficial effects on longevity and health (77). The FDA recommends that before a drug can be considered for approval it must lead to a weight loss ≥ 5% more than that achieved by a placebo and be statistically significantly greater (73). Improvement in comorbidities, such as diabetes, hypertension, hyperlipoproteinemia, respiratory insufficiency, sleep apnea, heart failure, and arthropathies, should be documented and used to evaluate the effectiveness of the drug. It is well documented that health risk factors associated with obesity are frequently ameliorated with as little as 5–10% weight loss (78). Ten per cent weight loss is a reasonable loss to expect with comprehensive weight loss programs, and that includes drug therapy where and when indicated. The weight loss slows down after the first few weeks when most overweight patients lose some water weight. It should be noted that the amount and the rate of weight loss is usually proportional to the starting weight of the person. People committed to lifestyle change and long follow-up have experienced much greater loss and have been able to maintain it; however, these are the exceptions. Most people regain all or part of their weight because they frequently stop treating their disease. The failure to maintain weight loss is in part a result of failure to continue treatment.

Few patients treated with drugs reach their goal weight and almost nobody reaches their "ideal" weight. The focus of the treatment should be on improving the physical and mental health of the patient and not on achieving an unrealistic dream weight (79). It is important to explain to the patients that obesity is a chronic condition and that weight management is a lifelong process.

SUGGESTIONS FOR THE USE OF OBESITY DRUGS

Recidivism is a more significant problem in obesity than in other chronic diseases. There is a strong feeling among practitioners and scientists treating and studying this disease that long-term—possible lifelong—therapy, including judicious use of drugs, may be indicated. The NHLBI, in their guidelines (75), suggest that an obesity medication may be taken indefinitely if it continues to be associated with weight loss and has no serious side-effects. This is with the understanding that treatment periods greater than 1 year have not been well studied and safety and efficacy must be continually monitored.

Recommended starting doses for more commonly used drugs are listed in Table 5-1 (46). Maximum doses are also listed. These drugs not infrequently have side-effects and lower starting doses may obviate some of them; tachyphylaxis may develop to lessen some of the other side-effects. It is recommended that obesity treatment be started with lowest possible effective dose and the adverse effects (if any) be carefully monitored. At every clinic visit, patients should be shown a list of possible serious drug-related side-effects and patients should be asked to check whether any of these apply. This practice may result in overestimating the prevalence of adverse effects; however, it might be better to exaggerate the adverse effects than to miss them. If the adverse effects are serious and life-threatening, or intolerable, the drug should be withdrawn. In cases where the adverse effects are serious but not life-threatening, dosage may be reduced under extreme vigilance, the drug may be changed, or the drug treatment may be stopped completely. Some adverse effects may decrease in intensity (or cease) over time. Weight loss progress should be considered if the adverse effects of a drug are mild or absent. Drug dosage need not be increased if the weight loss is satisfactory (≥1 lb week). Compliance with other components of the program, such as diet and lifestyle modification, should be ascertained if the weight loss is <1 lb for at least two consecutive weeks. Drug dosage may be increased if the weight loss is slow or unsatisfactory. Increase in drug dosage should be in small increments. Additional caution and monitoring for adverse effects should be exercised whenever a drug dosage is increased. Generally, the increased drug dosage should be reduced to previous levels if no additional weight loss is obtained.

The possibility of potential adverse effects of an obesity drug warrants screening of potential responders and non-responders to the drug treatment. To minimize the risk of adverse effects, drugs could be discontinued for the potential non-responders if they could be identified early during the treatment. Various predictors of drug-induced weight loss have been suggested. The package insert for dexfenfluramine recommended re-evaluation and possible discontinuation of the drug for patients losing >1.81 kg (4 lb) in the first month of treatment based on studies carried out by the manufacturer. The cut-off of a 4-lb weight loss in the first month of treatment was used widely by physicians to determine non-responders to fen–phen combination treatment. This criterion has become the standard for evaluating the response to most antiobesity drugs (76). However, a recent analysis by Dhurandhar et al (80) of weight loss response of 975 patients to phentermine and fenfluramine treatment showed that, in the total sample, first month weight loss highly correlated with percentage reduction in body mass index after 6 months of treatment. However, about 98% of the responders to the treatment (who lost >4 lb in the first month) had a weight reduction of 5% or greater in 6 months and 76% of the non-responders (who lost <4 lb in the first month) had met or exceeded the NAASO criteria for the success of a drug treatment (≥5% weight loss). Even the adverse effects after 6 months of treatment and the dropout rates after 1 year of treatment were not significantly different for non-responders vs. responders. This study indicated that although the first month weight loss predicted the long-term response to fen–phen treatment, it was inadequate in identifying the non-responders and may unnecessarily preclude potential beneficiaries of the treatment. A good criterion to identify non-responders early in the drug treatment remains to be defined.

RESULTS OF DRUG TREATMENT OF OBESITY

Single Drug Trials

Criteria for patient selection, as well as approaches and skills of physicians conducting studies and treatment programs associated with drug therapy are quite variable and make evaluation of results difficult to interpret. Most clinical trials have used single drug therapy. A review of over 200 studies by Scoville in 1976 revealed that the drugs available at that time were associated with approximately 0.5 lb/week greater weight loss than with placebo (81). Silverstone (32) reached similar conclusions when comparing short-term results from different agents.

Long-term studies that have evaluated obesity drugs for longer than 1 year are limited in number. Goldstein and Potvin (82) found only nine studies that had followed subjects for 1 year or more (Table 5-3). As seen in Table 5-3, with the exception of fluoxetine, longer term weight loss ranged from about 5 kg to about 14 kg and most of the drugs produced better weight loss than placebo. Even the placebo weight losses in several studies were very good, demonstrating that both groups underwent standard obesity therapy with diet, exercise, and behavioral therapy, which contributed to the weight loss observed. For example, mazindol produced the largest weight losses (14.2 kg) seen with a single agent in the review (82) but the large weight loss in the placebo group (10.2 kg) suggests that the behavioral component was very effective in this study.

Fluoxetine produced good weight loss over the first 6 months of treatment, although weight regain occurs thereafter and 1 year weight was not different between the placebo and experimental groups in 8 of 10 studies reported in a summary paper by Goldstein et al (83). Two sites that

Table 5-3 Long-Term Clinical Trials with Antiobesity Drugs

Antiobesity Drug	1 Year Weight Loss (kg)	
	Placebo	Active Agent
Diethylpropion	−10.5	−8.9
Mazindol	−10.2	−14.2
	−	−12.0
Fenfluramine	−4.5	−8.7
Dexfenfluramine	−7.2	−9.8
	−2.7	−5.7
	−4.6	−5.2
Fluoxetine	+0.6	−13.9
	−4.5	−8.2
	−1.5	−2.3
Sibutramine	−1.8	−6.0
Orlistat	−5.8	−8.8

included strong behavioral programs were able to obtain significant weight loss at 1 year (42,84).

Sibutramine, the latest centrally acting obesity drug approved by the FDA, produced weight losses of about 7–10 kg in a dose-dependent manner (85,86). Weight loss is very rapid in the first 12 weeks of treatment but does continue through 24 weeks of treatment. Treatment with sibutramine has been shown to reduce many of the risk factors associated with obesity such as cholesterol, triglycerides, and low-density lipoproteins (LDL), but reduction in blood pressure was noted to be less than with placebo with similar weight loss. Blood pressure and heart rate may actually increase in some patients and must be monitored closely, especially early in therapy. Patients should be very carefully followed-up and the medications should be stopped if weight loss is not satisfactory or if blood pressure rises.

Orlistat produces about 10% loss of initial body weight compared to about 6% weight loss in the placebo group (87). First year weight loss for the orlistat-treated group in a double-blind placebo-controlled trial (88) was 8.76 kg compared to 5.81 kg in the placebo group ($P < 0.001$). Subjects of this trial continuing to receive the drug for 2 years had significantly less weight regain in the second year compared to the placebo group. The orlistat group had improvement in fasting LDL-cholesterol and insulin levels. In another trial, 729 obese patients losing >8% of their body weight on hypo-caloric diet were treated with orlistat (30, 60, or 120 mg three times a day), or placebo, for 1 year (48). After 1 year, the sub-jects treated with 120 mg orlistat regained significantly less weight than the placebo group (32.8 vs. 58.7%, $P < 0.001$). Another study reported that orlistat treatment for 2 years promoted weight loss and minimized weight regain, im-proved lipid profile, blood pressure, and quality of life (49).

Combination Treatment

The combination of fenfluramine, a serotonin agonist, and phentermine, an adrenergic agonist, was first reported in 1984 by Weintraub et al (43). Weintraub et al (29) next per-formed a 4-year follow-up study that generated an enormous amount of publicity and changed the perception of the use of drugs for obesity. Although the combination of phenter-mine with fenfluramine or dexfenfluramine had a sudden demise when valvulopathy was reported in 1998, the com-bination was a highly effective drug regimen for weight loss. The fen–phen regimen popularized the concept of using more than one drug for treating obesity. The regimen also demonstrated that two drugs could be used in smaller than usual doses, minimizing adverse effects while enhancing the weight loss effect of the drugs.

The use of fluoxetine (20–60 mg/day) in combination with phentermine (18.75–37.5 mg/day) for 6-month periods produced significant weight loss (45). Whether longer periods of use of this combination will alleviate the regain noted with fluoxetine alone has not been studied to date.

Drug combinations such as ephedrine, caffeine, with or without aspirin, have produced weight losses that are as good as any drugs reported to date. Toubro et al (36) com-pared placebo, ephedrine alone, caffeine alone, and the combination of ephedrine and caffeine over a period of 24 weeks in 180 subjects. The combination of ephedrine and caffeine produced weight loss of about 16 kg at 24 weeks. Of the initial 180 subjects, 99 were followed for another 26 weeks in an open label study. Weight loss persisted for as long as the drugs were taken. This combination opened the door for further studies of combination drug therapy or stepwise therapy as an option for treating obesity. It is to be hoped that combination drug therapy with less significant or more tolerable side-effects will be developed in the future.

A COMPREHENSIVE WEIGHT MANAGEMENT PROGRAM

Obesity drugs should be only one part of a comprehensive program that includes dietary alterations, and increased physical activity; that is, alteration of behavior to attain a healthier lifestyle. A detailed description of the guidelines to set up an outpatient drug treatment program are published by Dhurandhar et al (89–91). These guidelines include special considerations for the patients, staff recruitment, clinic layout, and for the treatment itself. This article also deals with various related issues, such as dealing with the adverse reactions of obesity drugs, insurance issues, frequency of visits, and group therapy vs. single patient format.

Because obesity is a chronic condition, education of patients is critical. Physicians may not have the time needed to educate the patients extensively. Several guidelines suggest that obesity drug treatment be conducted by a health care team that includes a physician and one or more allied health professionals, such as a dietitian, nurse, exercise physiologist, psychologist, or counselor (74,76). Successful treatment of obesity will require increased awareness among patients and physicians, as well as the third party payees, that obesity is a chronic disease.

Reasonable and realistic weight loss goals in the range of 10% of the starting weight must be emphasized. At the same time, patients should be encouraged by the fact that weight loss can vary tremendously, and their response and the rate of weight loss is hard to predict accurately. Maintenance of the weight lost is the most important component of a weight management program. During their lifetime, many obese individuals lose (and regain) hundreds of pounds of weight. Health care professionals as well as patients should realize that successful weight loss is only the beginning of the battle. Preventing weight regain is truly the difficult aspect of weight management. Obesity drugs are currently used for producing weight loss. It is hoped that future research discovers drugs that could be used in the long term to prevent weight regain.

CONCLUSIONS

Obesity requires lifelong treatment. Drug therapy is in its infancy and long-term use of many of the drugs has not been adequately evaluated to date regarding either safety or efficacy. Weight loss with present medications is limited and usually plateaus in 6 months and after about 10% weight loss. There is evidence that patients may maintain the weight loss when the pharmacotherapy is continued in conjunction with a comprehensive weight management program. Weight management programs include physicians, dietitians, nurses, exercise physiologists, psychologists, and/or counselors.

Like any other drug, obesity drugs have a potential for adverse effects and minimizing the risk of such adverse effects should be a major concern. Drug therapy should be reserved for those patients with medically significant obesity with a favorable benefit:risk ratio. Candidates for drug treatment should be carefully screened. Careful follow-up and continuous assessment for efficacy and appearance of side-effects is mandatory.

A well-grounded weight management program including appropriate use of drugs and surgical referral capability allows the obese patient the best opportunity to obtain and retain a significant healthy weight loss.

REFERENCES

1. Bessesen D, Faggini R. Recently identified peptides involved in the regulation of body weight. Semin Oncol 1998; 25 (suppl 6): 28–32.

2. Bray G. Peptides and food intake: nutrient intake is modulated by peripheral peptide administration. Obes Res 1995; 3 (suppl 4): 569S–572S.

3. Gura T. Uncoupling proteins provide new clue to obesity causes. Science 1998; 280: 1369–1370.

4. Leibowitz S. Brain peptides and obesity: pharmacologic treatment. Obes Res 1995; 3 (suppl 4): 573S–589S.

5. Kuczmarski RJ, Carroll MD, Flegal KM, Troiano RP. Varying body mass index cut-off points to describe overweight prevalence among US adults: NHANES III (1988–1994). Obes Res 1997; 5: 542–549.

6. Kuczmarski RJ, Flegal KM, Campbell SM, Johnson CL. Increasing prevalence of overweight among US adults. JAMA 1994, 272: 205–211.

7. Balleisen L, Bailey J, Epping PH, Schulte H, van de Loo J. Epidemiological study on factor VII, factor VIII and fibrinogen in an industrial population. Thromb Haemost 1985; 54: 475–479.

8. Hubert HH, Feinliet M, McNamara PM, Costelli WA. Obesity as an independent risk factor for cardiovascular disease: a 26 year follow-up of participants in the Framingham Heart Study. Circulation 1983; 67: 968–977.

9. Park JJ, Swan PD. Effects of obesity and regional adiposity on the QT interval in women. Int J Obes 1997; 21: 1104–1110.

10. Alder M, Schaffner F. Fatty liver hepatitis and cirrhosis in obese patients. Am J Med 1979; 67: 811–816.

11. Rose M, Eliakin R, Bar-Ziv Y, Vromen A, Rachmilewitz D. Abdominal wall hernias: the value of computed tomography diagnosis in the obese patient. J Clin Gastroenterol 1994; 19: 94–96.

12. Wilson LJ, Ma W, Hirschowitz BI. Association of obesity with hiatal hernia and esophagitis. Am J Gastroenterol 1999; 94: 2840–2844.

13. Sugerman HJ, DeMaria EJ, Felton WL, Nakatsuka M, Sismanis A. Increased intra-abdominal pressure and cardiac filling pressures in obesity-associated pseudomotor cerebri. Neurology 1997; 49: 507–511.

14. Kasiske BL. Renal disease in patients with massive obesity. Arch Intern Med 1986; 146: 1105–1109.

15. Wesson DE, Kurtzman NA, Frommer JP. Massive obesity and nephrotic proteinaria with normal renal biopsy. Nephron 1985; 40: 235–237.

16. Bray, G. Health hazards associated with overweight. In: Bray GA, ed. Contemporary diagnosis and management of obesity. Newton, PA: Handbooks in Health Care, 1998; 68–103.

17. Kissebah A, Freedman DS, Peiris AN. Health risks of obesity. Med Clin North Am 1989; 73: 111–138.

18. Gross T, Sokol RJ, King KC. Obesity in pregnancy: risks and outcomes. Obstet Gynecol 1980; 56: 446–450.
19. Pasulka PS, Bistrian BR, Benotti PN, Blackburn GL. The risks of surgery in obese patients. Ann Intern Med 1986; 104: 540.
20. Connolly HM, Crary JL, McGoon MD, et al. Valvular heart disease associated with fenfluramine–phentermine. N Engl J Med 1997; 337: 581–588.
21. Kerman WN, Viscoli CM, Brass LM, Broderick JP, Brott T, et al. Phenylpropanolamine and the risk of hemorrhagic stroke. N Engl J Med 2000; 343: 1826–1832.
22. Sahu A, Kalra PS, Kalra SP. Food deprivation in ingestion induce reciprocal changes in neuropeptide Y concentrations in paraventricular nucleus. Peptides 1988; 9: 83–86.
23. Jung RT, Shetty PS, James WPT. Nutritional effects on thyroid and catacholamine metabolism. Clin Sci 1980; 58: 183–191.
24. Sclafani A. Animal models of obesity: classification and characterization. Int J Obes 1984; 8: 491–508.
25. Campfield LA, Smith FJ, Burn P. Strategies and potential targets for obesity treatment. Science 1998; 280: 1383–1387.
26. Broeder CE, Burrhus KA, Svanevik LS, Wilmore JH. The effect of either high intensity resistance or endurance training on resting metabolic rate. Am J Clin Nutr 1992; 55: 802–810.
27. Wadden TA, Vogt RA, Foster GD, Anderson DA. Exercise and the maintenance of weight loss: 1-year follow-up of a controlled clinical trial. J Consult Clin Psychol 1998; 66: 429–433.
28. Atkinson RL, Blank RC, Schumacher D, Dhurandhar NV, Ritch DL. Long-term drug treatment of obesity in a private practice setting. Obes Res 1997; 5: 578–586.
29. Weintraub M. Long-term weight control. The National Heart, Lung and Blood Institute Funded Multimodal Intervention Study. Clin Pharmacol Ther 1992; 51: 581–646.
30. Guy-Grand B, Apfelbaum M, Crepaldi G, Gries A, Lefebvre P, Turner P. International trial of long-term dexfenfluramine in obesity. Lancet 1989; 2: 1142–1145.
31. Levitsky DA, Troiano R. Metabolic consequences of fenfluramine for the control of body weight. Am J Clin Nutr 1992; 55: 167S–172S.
32. Silverstone T. Appetite suppressants: a review. Drugs 1992; 43: 820–836.
33. Wurtman JJ, Wurtman RJ, Reynolds S, Tsay R, Chew B. Fenfluramine suppresses snack intake among carbohydrate cravers but not among non-carbohydrate cravers. Int J Eat Disord 1987; 6: 687–699.

34. Blundell JE, Lawton CL, Halford JCG. Serotonin, eating behavior, and fat intake. Obes Res 1995; 3 (suppl 3): 471S–476S.
35. Daly PA, Krieger DR, Dulloo AG, Young JB, Landsberg L. Ephedrine, caffeine and aspirin: safety and efficacy for treatment of human obesity. Int J Obes 1993; 17 (suppl 1): S73–S78.
36. Toubro S, Astrup AV, Breum L, Quaade F. Safety and efficacy of long-term treatment with ephedrine, caffeine, and an ephedrine/caffeine mixture. Int J Obes 1993; 17 (suppl 1) S69–S72.
37. Liu YL, Toubro S, Astrup A, Stock MJ. Contribution of β3-adrenoceptor activation to ephedrine-induced thermogenesis in humans. Int J Obes 1995; 19: 678–685.
38. Stock MJ. Potential for β3-adrenoceptor agonists in the treatment of obesity. Int J Obes 1996; 20 (suppl 4): 4–5.
39. Troiano RP, Levitsky DA, Kalkwarf HJ. Effect of dl-fenfluramine on thermic effect of food in humans. Int J Obes 1990; 14: 647–655.
40. Schutz Y, Munger R, Deriaz O, Jequier E. Effect of dexfenfluramine on energy expenditure in man. Int J Obes 1992; 16 (suppl 3): S61–S66.
41. Griffiths RR, Brady JV, Bradford LD. Predicting the abuse liability of drugs with animal drug self-administration procedures: psychomotor stimulants and hallucinogens. Adv Behav Pharm 1979; 2: 163–208.
42. Darga LL, Carroll-Michals L, Botsford SJ, Lucas CP. Fluoxetine's effect on weight loss in obese subjects. Am J Clin Nutr 1991; 54: 321–325.
43. Weintraub M, Hasday JD, Mushlin AI, Lockwood DH. A double-blind clinical trial in weight control: use of fenfluramine and phentermine alone and in combination. Arch Intern Med 1984; 144: 1143–1148.
44. Spitz AF, Schumacher D, Blank RC, Dhurandhar NV, Atkinson RL. Safety and metabolic changes during long-term pharmacologic treatment of morbid obesity: a community based study. Endocr Pract 1997; 3: 269–275.
45. Dhurandhar NV, Atkinson RL. Comparison of serotonin agonists in combination with phentermine for treatment of obesity. FASEB J 1996; 10: A561.
46. Bray G. Drug treatment of overweight. In: Bray GA, ed. Contemporary diagnosis and management of obesity handbook. Newton, PA: Handbooks in Health Care, 1998: 246–273.
47. Mills, K. Serotonin syndrome. Am Fam Physician 1995; October: 1475–1482.
48. Hill JO, Hauptman J, Anderson JW, Fuijoka K, O'Neil PM, Smith DK, Zavoral JH, Arone LJ. Orlistat, a lipase inhibitor,

for weight maintenance after conventional dieting: 1-y study. Am J Clin Nutr 1999; 69: 1108–1116.

49. Rossner S, Sjostrom L, Noack R, Meinders E, Noseda G (European Orlistat Obesity Study Group). Weight loss, weight maintenance and improved cardiovascular risk factors after 2 years treatment with orlistat for obesity. Obes Res 2000; 8: 49–61.

50. Wolever TM, Chiasson JL, Josse RG, Hunt JA, et al. Small weight loss on long-term acarbose therapy with no change in dietary pattern or nutrient intake of individual with low insulin-dependent diabetes. Int J Obes 1997; 21: 756–763.

51. Pittler MH, Abbot NC, Harkness EF, Ernst E. Randomized double-blind trial of Chitosan for body weight reduction. Eu J Clin Nutr 1999; 53: 379–381.

52. Horton TJ, Geissler CA. Postprandial thermogenesis with ephedrine, caffeine and aspirin in lean predisposed obese and obese women. Int J Obes 1996; 20: 91–97.

53. Haller CA, Benowitz NL. Adverse cardiovascular and central nervous system events associated with dietary supplements containing ephedra alkaloids. N Engl J Med 2000; 343: 1833–1838.

54. Atkinson RL. Conjugated linoleic acid for altering body composition and treating obesity. In: Yurowecz M, et al. (eds). Advances in conjugated linoleic acid, Vol 1. Champaign, IL: AOCS Press, 1999: 348–353.

55. Ostrowska E, Muralitharan M, Cross RF, Bauman DE, Dunshea FR. Dietary conjugated linoleic acids increase lean tissue and decrease fat deposition in growing pigs. J Nutr 1999; 129: 2037–2042.

56. Dulloo AG, Duret C, Rohrer D, Girardier L, et al. Effect of a green tea extract rich in catechin polyphenols and caffeine in increasing 24-hour energy expenditure and fat oxidation in humans. Am J Clin Nutr 1999; 70: 1040–1045.

57. Heymsfield SB, Allison DB, Vasselli JR, Pietrobelli A, Greenfield D, Nunez C. Garcinia cambogia (hydroxy citric acid) as a potential antiobesity agent: a randomized controlled trial. JAMA 1998; 280: 1596–1600.

58. Jaedig S, Henningsen N. Increased metabolic rate in obese women after ingestion of potassium, magnesium and phosphate-enriched orange juice or injection of ephedrine. Int J Obes 1991; 15: 429–436.

59. Jaedig S, Lindgarde F, Arborelius M. Increased postprandial energy expenditure in obese women after peroral potassium and magnesium phosphate. Miner Electrolyte Metab 1994; 20: 147–152.

60. Fontgonne A, Andre P, Eschwege E. Biguanides and the prevention of the risk of obesity. Diabetes Metab 1991; 17 (1 Pt 2): 249–254.

61. Paolisso G, Amato L, Eccellente R, Gambardella A, et al. Effect of metformin on food intake in obese subjects. Eur J Clin Invest 1998; 28 (6): 44–46.
62. Pasquali R, Gambineri A, Biscotti D, Vicennati V, et al. Effect of long-term treatment with metformin added to hypocaloric diet and body composition, fat distribution and androgen and insulin levels in abdominally obese women with and without the polycystic ovary syndrome. J Clin Endocrin Metab 2000; 85: 2767–2774.
63. Doose DR, Walker SA, Gisclon LG, Nayak RK. Single dose pharmacokinetics and effect of food on the bioavailability of topiramate, a novel antiepileptic drug. J Clin Pharmacol 1996; 36: 884–891.
64. Perucca E. A pharmacological and clinical review on topiramate, a new antiepileptic drug. Pharmacol Res 1997; 35: 241–256.
65. Gordon A, Price LH. Mood stabilization and weight loss with topiramate [Letter]. Am J Psychiatry 1999; 156: 968–969.
66. Shapira NA, Goldsmith TD, McElroy SL. Treatment of binge eating disorders with topiramate: a clinical case study. J Clin Psychiatry 2000; 61: 368–372.
67. Osburne RC, Myers EA, Rodbard D, et al. Adaptation to hypocaloric feeding: physiological significance of the fall in T3 as measured by the pulse wave arrival time. Metabolism 1983; 32: 9–13.
68. Stockholm KH, Andersen T, Lindgreen P. Low serum free T3 concentrations in post obese patients previously treated with very low calorie diet. Int J Obes 1987; 11: 85–89.
69. Montzoros C. The role of leptin in human obesity and disease: a review of current evidence. Ann Intern Med 1999; 130: 671–680.
70. Considine RV, Sinha MK, Heiman ML, Kriauciunas A, Stephens TW, Nyce MR, Ohannesian JP, Marco CC, McKee LJ, Bauer TL, Caro JF. Serum immunoreactive-leptin concentrations in normal-weight and obese humans. N Engl J Med 1996; 334: 292–295.
71. Heymsfield SB, Greenberg AS, Fujioka K, Dixon RM, Kushner R, Hunt T, Lubina JA, Patane J, Self B, Hunt P, McCamish M. Recombinant leptin for weight loss in obese and lean adults: a randomized, controlled dose escalation trial. JAMA 1999; 282: 1568–1575.
72. National Institutes of Health (NIH) National Taskforce on the prevention and treatment of obesity: long-term pharmacotherapy in the management of obesity. JAMA 1996; 276: 1907–1915.
73. Food and Drug Administration. Guidance for the clinical evaluation of weight control drugs. Rockville, MD: Food and Drug Administration, 1996.

74. Pi-Sunyer XF. Guidelines for the approval and use of antiobesity drugs. Obes Res 1995; 3: 473–478.
75. National Heart, Lung and Blood Institute. Clinical guidelines on the identification, evaluation, and treatment of overweight and obesity in adults: the evidence report. Obes Res 1998; 6 (suppl 2) 51S–183S.
76. Shape Up America! and American Obesity Association. Guidance for treatment of adult obesity. Bethesda, MD: Shape Up America! 1996.
77. Allison DB, Zannolli R, Faith MS, Heo M, et al. Weight loss increases and fat loss decreases all cause mortality rate. Int J Obes 1999; 23: 603–611.
78. Kanders BS, Blackburn GL. Reducing primary risk factors by therapeutic weight loss. In: Wadden TA, Van Itallie TB, eds. Treatment of the seriously obese patient. New York: Guilford Press, 1992: 213–230.
79. Foster GD, Wadden TA, Vogt RA, Brewer G. What is a reasonable weight loss? Patient's expectations and evaluations of obesity treatment outcomes. J Consult Clin Psychol 1997; 65: 79–85.
80. Dhurandhar NV, Blank RC, Schumacher D, Atkinson RL. Initial weight loss as a predictor of response to antiobesity drugs. Int J Obes 1999; 23: 1333–1336.
81. Scoville BA. Review of amphetamine-like drugs by the Food and Drug Administration. In: Bray GA, ed. Obesity in perspective. Washington, DC: Fogarty International Center for Advanced Studies in Health Sciences Series on Preventive Medicine II, US Government Printing Office, 1976: 441–443.
82. Goldstein DJ, Potvin JH. Long-term weight loss: the effect of pharmacologic agents. Am J Clin Nutr 1994; 60: 647–657.
83. Goldstein DJ, Rampey AH Jr, Dornseif BE, Levine LR, Potvin JH, Fludzinski LA. Fluoxetine: a randomized clinical trial in the maintenance of weight loss. Obes Res 1993; 1: 92–98.
84. Marcus MD, Wing RR, Ewing L, Kern E, McDermott M, Gooding W. A double-blind, placebo-controlled trial of fluoxetine plus behavior modification in the treatment of obese binge-eaters and non-binge-eaters. Am J Psychiatry 1990; 147: 876–881.
85. Bray GA, Ryan DH, Gordon D, Heidingsfelder S, Cerise F, Wilson K. A double-blind randomized placebo-controlled trial of sibutramine. Obes Res 1996; 4: 263–270.
86. Ryan DH, Kaiser P, Bray GA. Sibutramine: a novel new agent for obesity treatment. Obes Res 1995; 3 (suppl 4): 553S–559S.
87. Sjostrom L, Rissanen A, Andersen T, Boldrin M, Golay A, Koppeschaar HP, Krempf M. Randomized placebo controlled trial of orlistat for weight loss and prevention of weight regain in obese patients. Lancet 1998; 352: 167–172.

88. Davidson MH, Hauptman J, DiGirolamo M, Foreyt JP, Halsted CH, Heber D, Heimburger DC, Lucas CP, Robbins DC, Chung J, Heymsfeld SB. Weight control and risk factor reduction in obese subjects treated for 2 years with orlistat: a randomized controlled trial. JAMA 1999; 281: 235–242.
89. Dhurandhar NV, Atkinson RL. Drug treatment of obesity: guidelines for an outpatient program. J Am Soc Bariatric Physicians 1997; Summer: 18–23.
90. Dhurandhar N, Allison D. The pharmacologic treatment of obesity. Econ Neuroscience 2000; August: 42–52.
91. Dhurandhar NV, Allison DB. Algorithm for pharmacological treatment of obesity. Primary Psychiatry 2001; 8: 63–78.

Chapter 6

Surgery for Morbid Obesity

Harvey J. Sugerman, Eric J. DeMaria,
and John M. Kellum

Severely obese patients suffer from a multitude of medical
problems, some of which may be life-threatening and others
that severely limit the individual's ability to lead productive
lives, giving rise to the term "morbid obesity" (Table 6-1).
Premature death is much more common in severely obese
individuals. Comorbid conditions that can be associated
with an earlier mortality include an increased incidence of
coronary artery disease, hypertension, impaired cardiac
function, adult onset diabetes mellitus, obesity hypoventilation and/or sleep apnea syndromes (known collectively as
the Pickwickian syndrome), venous stasis disease and hyper-
coagulability leading to an increased risk of pulmonary
embolus, and necrotizing panniculitis. Of special importance to surgeons is the increased difficulty in recognizing
peritonitis in a morbidly obese patient. Severe obesity is also
associated with an increased risk of uterine, breast, prostate,
and colon carcinoma. A number of obesity-related problems
are not life-threatening but can cause significant physical or
psychological disability, including degenerative osteoarthritis, pseudotumor cerebri, cholecystitis, skin infections,
chronic venous stasis ulcers, stress and/or urge overflow

Table 6-1 Morbidity of Severe Obesity

Central obesity
Metabolic complications (Syndrome X)
   Non-insulin dependent diabetes (adult onset/type 2)
   Hypertension
   Dyslipidemia: elevated triglycerides, cholesterol
   Cholelithiasis, cholecystitis
Increased intra-abdominal pressure
   Stress overflow urinary incontinence
   Gastroesophageal reflux
   Venous disease: thrombophlebitis, venous stasis ulcers
     Pulmonary embolism
   Obesity hypoventilation syndrome
   Nephrotic syndrome
   Hernias (incisional, inguinal)
   Pre-eclampsia
Respiratory insufficiency of obesity (Pickwickian syndrome)
   Obesity hypoventilation syndrome
   Obstructive sleep apnea syndrome
Cardiovascular dysfunction
   Coronary artery disease
   Increased complications after coronary bypass surgery
   Heart failure subsequent to:
     Left ventricular concentric hypertrophy—hypertension
     Left ventricular eccentric hypertrophy—obesity
Right ventricular hypertrophy—pulmonary failure
     Prolonged Q-T interval with sudden death
Sexual hormone dysfunction
   Amenorrhea, hypermenorrhea
   Stein–Leventhal syndrome: hirsutism, ovarian cysts
   Infertility
   Endometrial carcinoma
   Breast carcinoma
Other carcinomas: colon, renal cell, prostate
Infectious complications
   Difficulty recognizing peritonitis
   Necrotizing pancreatitis
   Necrotizing subcutaneous infections
   Wound infections, dehiscence
Pseudotumor cerebri (idiopathic intracranial hypertension)
Degenerative osteoarthritis
   Feet, ankles, knees, hips, back, shoulders
Psychosocial impairment
Decreased employability, work discrimination

urinary incontinence, gastroesophageal reflux, sex hormone imbalance with dysmenorrhea, hirsutism, infertility, as well as an increased incidence of all types of hernias: incisional, inguinal and umbilical. Many of these individuals suffer from severe psychological and social disability, including marked prejudice regarding employment.

CENTRAL OBESITY SYNDROME X VERSUS INCREASED INTRA-ABDOMINAL PRESSURE

There are data documenting that central, or android, obesity is much more dangerous than peripheral, or gynoid, obesity. This is thought to be secondary to increased visceral fat metabolism leading to hyperglycemia, diabetes, and insulin-induced sodium reabsorption, leading to hypertension. This combination of metabolic problems is known as "Syndrome X"[1,2]. We have found that central obesity also is associated with a marked increase in intra-abdominal pressure (Figure 6-1), as estimated from urinary bladder pressure [3]. Bladder pressures in patients with central obesity, as measured by sagittal abdominal diameter, are often as high, or higher, than those in patients with an acute abdominal compartment syndrome where it is recommended that they undergo abdominal decompression. Increased intra-abdominal pressure may lead to venous stasis ulcers, obesity hypoventilation syndrome, gastroesophageal reflux, increased intracranial pressure associated with pseudotumor cerebri and incisional hernias. The urinary bladder pressure was found to be significantly higher in patients with three or more comorbidity problems per patient than those with two or less (Figure 6-2).

SURGERY FOR OBESITY

Although many individuals can lose weight successfully through dietary manipulation, the incidence of recidivism in the morbidly obese approaches 95% [4]. In 1991, a National Institutes of Health (NIH) Consensus Conference stated that

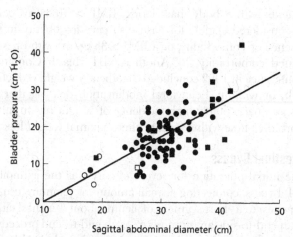

Figure 6-1 Correlation between urinary bladder pressure and sagittal abdominal diameter in 84 morbidly obese patients (● women; ■ men *f*) and 5 "control" non-obese patients (○ women; □ men) with ulcerative colitis, r = +0.67, *P* < 0.0001. (From Sugerman al (3) with permission.)

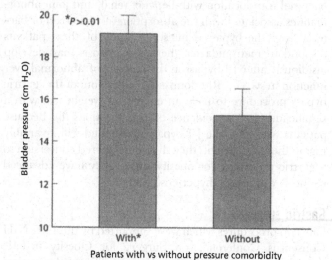

Figure 6-2 Increased urinary bladder pressure in patients with three or more than those with two, one, or no probable or possible pressure-related comorbidity problems. (From Sugerman et al (3) with permission.)

patients with a body mass index (BMI) > $40 \, \text{kg/m}^2$ could be considered eligible for gastric surgery for obesity in the absence of comorbidity, or a BMI > $35 \, \text{kg/m}^2$ with obesity-related comorbidity (5). Another NIH Health Consensus Conference in 1992 concluded that dietary weight reduction with, or without, behavioral modification or drug therapy has an unacceptably high incidence of weight regain in the morbidly obese within 2 years after maximal weight loss (6).

Intestinal Bypass

The initial operation for severe obesity was the jejunoileal (J-I) bypass, connecting a small amount of jejunum (usually 8 inches) to a short segment of ileum (about 4 inches) either as an end-to-side anastomosis or as an end-to-end procedure with the bypassed intestine connected to the colon. Although effective for weight loss, this procedure is associated with a number of complications, which can be divided into meta-bolic, nutritional, and electrolyte abnormalities or problems secondary to bacterial overgrowth in the bypassed, "blind-limb", intestine (7). This operation is a model of iatrogenic bacterial translocation with hepatic, renal, and joint abnor-malities associated with the absorption of endotoxin or bac-teria from the bypassed intestine. Many of these patients respond to metronidazole therapy. Cirrhosis may develop insidiously after J-I bypass in the absence of abnormal liver function tests (7). Randomized studies found the gastric bypass procedure to have an equivalent weight loss with a significantly lower incidence of complications (8). Because patients who have the J-I bypass dismantled will invariably regain their lost weight, they should be offered conversion to a gastric procedure for obesity, unless they have advanced cirrhosis with portal hypertension (9).

Gastric surgery

The two procedures which were supported by the 1991 NIH Consensus Conference on Surgery for Obesity include the gastric bypass (GBP) (10) (Figure 6-3) and the vertical banded (VBGP) (11) (Figure 6-4) or silastic ring gastroplasty. In a randomized prospective trial, it was found that GBP had a significantly greater weight loss than VBGP (Figure 6-5),

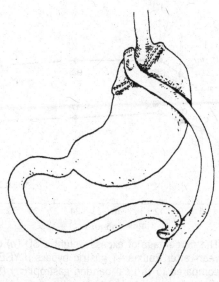

Figure 6-3 Roux-en-Y gastric bypass. (From Sugerman et al (10) with permission.)

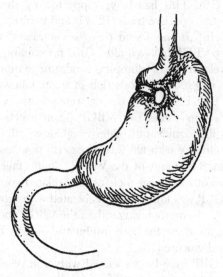

Figure 6-4 Vertical banded gastroplasty. (From Sugerman et al (10) with permission.)

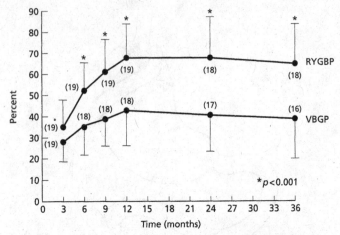

Figure 6-5 The percentage of excess weight ± SD (*n*) over 3 years after Roux-en-Y gastric bypass (RYGBP) compared to vertical banded gastroplasty (VBGP). (From Sugerman et al (10) with permission.)

which was especially true for patients who were addicted to sweets (10). This has been supported by three other randomized prospective trials (12–14) and two retrospective studies (15,16). It was found that "sweet eaters" did very poorly after VBGP but well after GBP, presumably because of the development of dumping syndrome symptoms following the ingestion of foods rich in sugar following GBP (10) (Table 6-2). Even when patients were selectively assigned to GBP ("sweets eaters") or VBGP ("non-sweets eaters"), there was still a significantly better weight loss with GBP and no loss of efficacy with all "sweets eaters" now assigned to GBP (Figure 6-6); many of the VBGP patients failed to lose enough weight to correct their obesity-related comorbidity (17). The GBP was found to be associated with significantly higher levels of enteroglucagon than the VBGP and a lower area under the curve for both insulin and glucose following 100 g of oral glucose (18).

The GBP may be associated with iron, vitamin B_{12}, and calcium deficiencies, which usually respond to oral

| Table 6-2 | Percentage Decrease in Excess Weight in Sweets Eaters vs. Non-Sweets Eaters with Gastric Bypass (GBP) vs. Vertical Banded Gastroplasty (VBGP). (From Sugerman et al (3) with permission.) |

Sweets Eaters	Non-Sweets Eaters
GBP	
(1) 69 ± 17 ⟨12⟩	67 ± 17 ⟨7⟩
(2) 62 ± 19 ⟨11⟩	75 ± 19 ⟨7⟩
(3) 59 ± 17 ⟨11⟩	71 ± 21 ⟨7⟩
P < 0.001	NS
VBGP	
(1) 36 ± 13 ⟨12⟩	57 ± 18 ⟨6⟩
(2) 35 ± 14 ⟨11⟩	53 ± 22 ⟨6⟩
(3) 32 ± 18 ⟨11⟩	50 ± 21 ⟨5⟩
P < 0.05	

supplementation (10,17). Rapid weight loss following surgery for obesity is associated with a 32% risk of gallstone formation which can be decreased to 2% with 300 mg prophylactic ursodiol taken twice daily for 6 months (19). Stomal stenosis or marginal ulcer may occur in approximately 12% of patients each, but usually respond to endoscopic balloon dilatation or antacid therapy, respectively (20). There are three potential spaces for internal herniation, which may have a normal upper gastrointestinal radiographic barium series and be very difficult to diagnose.

Three studies have shown that weight loss following GBP is long-lasting in the vast majority of patients, with the average weight loss at 2 years to be 66% of excess weight, 60% at 5 years and mid-50s at 5–10 years following surgery, an acceptable risk of complications and a mortality rate of ≤0.5% (15,21,22). Ten to 15% of patients will fail the

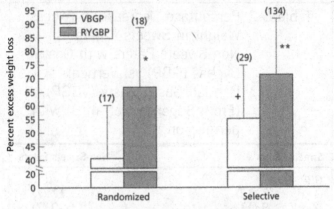

* P<0.001 Randomized RYGBP vs VBGP
** P<0.01 Selective RYGBP vs VBGP
+ Selective VBGP vs randomized VBGP

Figure 6-6 Percentage of excess weight loss at 2 years following selective assignment of sweets eaters to GBP and non-sweets eaters to VBGP as compared to random assignment. (From Sugerman et al (17) with permission.)

operation as defined by the loss of ≤40% of excess weight. Vertical banded gastroplasty may be associated with a high incidence of outlet stenosis, gastroesophageal reflux disease (GERD) or failed weight loss because of maladaptive eating behavior as many patients are unable to tolerate normal nutritious foods and become sweets or junk food eaters. Conversion to gastric bypass has had a low risk of morbidity and weight loss results equivalent to primary gastric bypass with correction of GERD symptoms (23,24). Patients who are superobese (BMI >50 kg/m^2) only lose one half of their excess weight at 2 years (17,25); lengthening the Roux-en-Y limb from 18 to 59 inches (45 to 150 cm) ("long-limb GBP") was found to increase their weight loss to two thirds of excess weight, without any apparent increased nutritional deficiencies (25).

All forms of horizontal gastroplasty have been found to have an unacceptable incidence of weight loss failure, as well as a high complication rate related to gastric leaks or splenic injury (26). There are several types of gastric banding procedures. Swedish studies found that gastric banding has an extremely variable and often inadequate weight loss as well as frequent mechanical problems associated with outlet obstruction. A more recent modification using a laparoscopic adjustable silicone gastric band may have more favorable results (27) but awaits convincing data from prospective studies and is currently under evaluation in the United States at seven medical centers before approval for generalized use can be provided by the Food and Drug Administration. Concerns with the procedure include risk of band erosion into the stomach, band slippage with outlet obstruction, esophageal dilatation and inadequate weight loss (28). Laparoscopic gastric bypass is a surgical *tour de force* that has become the procedure of choice at several institutions for patients with a BMI ≤50 kg/m², although several centers are performing the procedure for superobese patients (29,30). There appears to be an increased risk of an anastomotic leak, and possibly pulmonary embolism, with the laparoscopic approach. Most laparoscopic GBP centers place prophylactic drains which reduce the risk of an anastomotic leak. Because of the increased intra-abdominal pressure there is a high incidence (20%) of incisional hernia following a mid-line laparotomy incision (31); laparoscopic approaches will markedly reduce the risk of this complication.

Partial Biliopancreatic Bypass and Duodenal Switch Operations

A more radical procedure proposed for the treatment of severely obese patients is the partial biliopancreatic diversion which involves a subtotal gastrectomy leaving a 400-cc gastric pouch for the average obese patient and a 200-cc gastric pouch for the superobese patient (32). The distal small bowel is transected 250 cm proximal to the ileocecal valve and the proximal, bypassed bowel is anastomosed to the ileum 50 cm proximal to the ileocecal valve. This leaves a 200-cm "alimentary tract", a 300–400 cm "biliary tract" of bypassed intestine, and a 50-cm "common absorptive alimentary tract", where the ingested food mixes with bile and pancreatic juices for digestion and absorption. Thus, this is both a gastric restrictive and intestinal malabsorptive procedure. The biliopancreatic diversion has had excellent weight loss results and does not appear to be associated with the high incidence of bacterial overgrowth and translocation problems of the J-I bypass, as bile and pancreatic juices wash out the bypassed small intestine. However, the biliopancreatic diversion may be associated with severe protein-calorie malnutrition, necessitating hospitalization and total parenteral nutrition; frequent, foul-smelling steatorrheic stools which float leading to fat-soluble vitamin deficiencies and calcium loss secondary to chelation with fat, leading to severe osteoporosis. It is possible that patients in Italy, where the operation was developed, have fewer nutritional problems as their diet is high in complex carbohydrates (e.g. pasta) as compared to American patients whose diet is much higher in fat (e.g. fried foods, potato or corn chips). A randomized prospective trial using a much smaller stomach (50 cc) without gastric resection and a longer common absorptive intestinal tract (150 cm) in superobese patients, called a distal GBP, was associated with a much greater weight loss than a standard GBP, but had a 25% incidence of severe malnutrition necessitating conversion to the standard GBP (33). We currently reserve this type of distal GBP for superobese patients who fail a standard GBP and have severe obesity-related comorbidity (e.g. diabetes, Picwickian syndrome), recognizing that there will be a need for fat-soluble vitamin supplementation as well as a risk of severe malnutrition (33).

A modified malabsorptive procedure, known as the duodenal switch operation (34), has been developed with the hope that there will be less protein and fat-soluble vitamin malabsorption. This procedure involves wedge resection of the greater curvature of the stomach, division of the duodenum in the distal bulb and the ileum 250 cm proximal to the ileocecal valve with anastomosis of the proximal duodenal segment to the distal ileal segment; the distal end of the transected duodenum is oversewn as a duodenal stump. The proximal segment, which carries the biliary and pancreatic secretions, is anastomosed end-to-side for an enteroenterostomy 100 cm proximal to the ileocecal valve. It is not clear yet if this operation will prevent the protein malnutrition, calcium and fat-soluble vitamin deficiencies associated with a malabsorptive procedure.

SUMMARY

In conclusion, the gastric bypass has significantly better weight loss than the vertical banded or silastic ring gastroplasty, but may be associated with iron, vitamin B_{12}, and calcium deficiencies, which usually can be overcome with oral prophylaxis, as well as stomal stenosis or marginal ulcer which also usually respond to medical treatment. Horizontal gastroplasties have very high failure and complication rates and should no longer be performed. Gastric banding appears to have results similar to gastroplasty in addition to problems with outlet obstruction. The laparoscopic adjustable gastric band is currently under evaluation for the Food and Drug Administration for use in the United States but is a very popular procedure in Europe and Australia where more than 50,000 have been inserted, mostly laparoscopically. The "long-limb GBP" appears to be the procedure of choice for superobese patients. Biliopancreatic diversion, distal gastric bypass and, possibly, the duodenal switch operation provide excellent long-term weight loss but may cause severe protein-calorie malnutrition, fat-soluble vitamin deficiencies, and osteoporosis, especially in American patients.

Significant long-lasting weight loss follows gastric surgery for obesity and this loss of weight is associated with amelioration, or complete resolution, of the morbidity associated with severe obesity, including obstructive sleep apnea syndrome (35,36), obesity hypoventilation (35), gastroesophageal reflux (37,38), pseudotumor cerebri (39), systemic hypertension (40,41), hypercholesterolemia (42,43), cardiac dysfunction of obesity (44), type 2 diabetes (45), female sexual hormone dysfunction (46), chronic lower extremity joint and back pains (47), venous stasis ulcers (48),

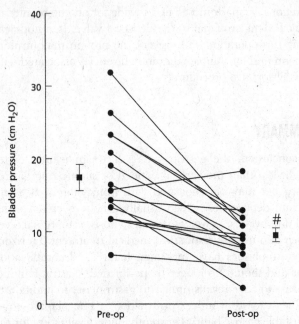

Figure 6-7 Urinary bladder pressure before and 1 year following gastric bypass induced loss of 69 ± 4% excess weight. (From Sugerman et al (51) with permission.)

urinary incontinence (49) and improves self-image and employability (50). The increased intra-abdominal pressure associated with an increased sagittal abdominal diameter in central obesity decreases significantly with surgically induced weight loss which is associated with improvement or resolution of intra-abdominal pressure related and non-related comorbidity (51) (Figure 6-7). It is not often that a surgeon can perform one operation and cure four or five diseases. Although insurance coverage for bariatric surgery can be a problem with some state Medicaid programs, as well as "Health Maintenance Organizations" (HMOs), inappropriate procedures in the morbidly obese would most likely be supported, such as lumboperitoneal shunts for pseudotumor cerebri, skin grafts (which usually will not take) for venous stasis ulcers, Nissen fundoplication for gastroesophageal reflux, and bladder suspension for stress and/or urge overflow urinary incontinence. It is tragic that patients with these severe comorbidities are prevented from having access to a procedure that may not only be life-saving but also markedly improve the quality of their lives. These HMOs seem to be more concerned with this year's financial "bottom line" than the ultimate cost of care over 5–10 years.

The Swedish Obesity Study (SOS) has found that surgically induced weight loss was associated with a significant decrease in type 2 diabetes, systemic hypertension, pulmonary dysfunction, and sick leave with enhanced tax returns from increased employability as compared to a matched group of controls who were managed by their primary care physicians (52–55). The East Carolina University group noted a significantly lower mortality in diabetic patients who underwent gastric bypass (6% at 9 years) as compared to patients who did not have bariatric surgery either because of the inability to obtain insurance coverage or for personal reasons (28% at 6 years) (56).

Gastric surgery for obesity mandates surgeons dedicated to the treatment of the morbidly obese, long-term follow-up with the assistance of dietitians to maximize dietary compliance and weight loss, as well as to prevent micronutrient deficiencies. The potential complications are significant; however, the surgeon who is aware of these problems can minimize the risks and be rewarded with a very grateful group of patients.

REFERENCES

1. Kissebah A, Vydelingum N, Murray R, et al. Relation of body fat distribution to metabolic complications of obesity. J Clin Endocrinol Metab 1982; 54: 254–257.
2. Kvist A, Chowdhury B, Grangard U, Tylen U, Sjostrom L. Total and visceral adipose tissue volumes derived from measurements with computed tomography in adult men and women: predictive equations. Am J Clin Nutr 1988; 48: 1351–1361.

3. Sugerman H, Windsor A, Bessos M, Wolfe M. Abdominal pressure, sagittal abdominal diameter and obesity co-morbidity. J Int Med 1997; 241: 71–79.
4. Johnson D, Drennick EJ. Therapeutic fasting in morbid obesity. Arch Intern Med 1977; 137: 1381–1382.
5. National Institutes of Health (NIH) Conference. Gastrointestinal surgery for severe obesity: Consensus Development Conference Panel. Ann Int Med 1991; 115: 956–961.
6. NIH Conference. Methods for voluntary weight loss and control: NIH Technology Assessment Conference Panel. Ann Int Med 1992; 116: 942–949.
7. Hocking MP, Duerson MC, O'Leary PJ, et al. Jejunoileal bypass for morbid obesity: late follow-up in 100 cases. N Engl J Med 1983; 308: 995–999.
8. Griffen WO, Young VL, Stevenson CC. A prospective comparison of gastric and jejunoileal bypass for morbid obesity. Ann Surg 1977; 186: 500–509.
9. Halverson JD, Gentry K, Wise L, et al. Reanastomosis after jejunoileal bypass. Surgery 1978; 84: 241–249.
10. Sugerman HJ, Starkey JV, Birkenhauer R. A randomized prospective trial of gastric bypass versus vertical banded gastroplasty for morbid obesity and their effects on sweets versus non-sweets eaters. Ann Surg 1987; 205: 613–624.
11. Mason EE. VBG: Effective treatment of uncontrolled obesity. Bull Am Coll Surg 1991; 76: 18–22.
12. MacLean LD, Rhode BM, Sampalis J, Forse RA. Results of the surgical treatment of obesity. Am J Surg 1993; 165: 155–160.
13. Howard L, Malone M, Michalek A, et al. Gastric bypass and vertical banded gastroplasty: a prospective randomized comparison and 5-year follow-up. Obes Surg 1995; 5: 55–60.
14. Capella JF, Capella RF. The weight reduction operation of choice: vertical banded gastroplasty or gastric bypass? Am J Surg 1996; 171: 74–79.
15. Yale CE. Gastric surgery for morbid obesity: complications and long-term weight control. Arch Surg 1989; 124: 941–946.
16. Kenler HA, Brolin RE, Cody RO. Changes in eating behavior after horizontal gastroplasty and Roux-en-Y gastric bypass. Am J Clin Nutr 1990; 52: 87–91.
17. Sugerman HJ, Londrey GL, Kellum JM, et al. Weight loss with vertical banded gastroplasty and Roux-en-Y gastric bypass for morbid obesity with selective versus random assignment. Am J Surg 1989; 157: 93–100.
18. Kellum J, Kuemmerle J, O'Dorisio T, et al. Gastrointestinal hormone responses to meals before and after gastric bypass

and vertical banded gastroplasty. Ann Surg 1990; 211: 763–771.

19. Sugerman HJ, Brewer WH, Shiffman ML, et al. A multicenter, placebo-controlled, randomized, double-blind, prospective trial of prophylactic ursodiol for the prevention of gallstone formation following gastric-bypass-induced rapid weight loss. Am J Surg 1995; 169: 91–97.
20. Sanyal AJ, Sugerman HJ, Kellum JM, Engle KM, Wolfe L. Stomal complications of gastric bypass: incidence and outcome of therapy. Am J Gastroenterol 1992; 87: 1165–1169.
21. Sugerman HJ, Kellum JM, Engle KM, et al. Gastric bypass for treating severe obesity. Am J Clin Nutr 1992; 55: 560S–566S.
22. Pories WJ, MacDonald KG, Morgan EJ, et al. Surgical treatment of obesity and its effects on diabetes: 10-yr follow-up. Am J Clin Nutr 1992; 55: 582S–585S.
23. Kim CH, Sarr MG. Severe reflux esophagitis after vertical banded gastroplasty for treatment of morbid obesity. Mayo Clin Proc 1992; 67: 33–35.
24. Sugerman HJ, Kellum JM, DeMaria EJ, Reines HD. Conversion of failed or complicated vertical banded gastroplasty to gastric bypass in morbid obesity. Am J Surg 1996; 171: 263–269.
25. Brolin RE, Kenler HA, Gorman JH, Cody RP. Long-limb gastric bypass in the superobese: a prospective randomized study. Ann Surg 1992; 215: 387–392.
26. Sugerman HJ, Wolper JL. Failed gastroplasty for morbid obesity: revised gastroplasty versus Roux-en-Y gastric bypass. Am J Surg 1984; 148: 331–336.
27. Belachew M, Legrand M, Vincent V, Lismonde M, LeDocte N, Deschamps V. Laparoscopic adjustable gastric banding. World J Surg 1998; 22: 955–963.
28. DeMaria EJ, Sugerman HJ, Meador JG, Doty JM, Kellum JM, Wolfe L, Szucs RA, Turner MA. High failure rate following laparoscopic adjustable silicone gastric banding for treatment of morbid obesity. Ann Surg 2001; 233: 809–818.
29. Wittgrove AC, Clark GW, Schubert KR. Laparoscopic gastric bypass, Roux-en-Y: the results in 500 patients with 5-year follow-up. Obes Surg 2000; 10: 233–239.
30. Schauer PR, Ikramuddin S, Gourash W, Ramanathan R, Luketich J. Outcomes after laparoscopic Roux-en-Y gastric bypass for morbid obesity. Ann Surg 2000; 232: 515–529.
31. Sugerman HJ, Kellum JM, Reines HD, DeMaria EJ, Newsome HH, Lowry JW. Greater risk of incisional hernia with morbidly obese than steroid dependent patients and low recurrence

with prefascial polypropylene mesh. Am J Surg 1966; 171: 80–84.

32. Scopinaro N, Gianetta D, Adami G, et al. Biliopancreatic diversion for obesity at eighteen years. Surgery 1996; 119: 261–268.

33. Sugerman HJ, Kellum JM, DeMaria EJ. Conversion of proximal to distal gastric bypass for failed gastric bypass for superobesity. J Gastrointest Surg 1997; 1: 517–525.

34. Lagace M, Marceau P, Marceau S, et al. Biliopancreatic diversion with a new type of gastrectomy: some previous conclusions revisited. Obes Surg 1995; 5: 411–418.

35. Sugerman HJ, Fairman RP, Sood RK, et al. Long-term effects of gastric surgery for treating respiratory insufficiency of obesity. Am J Clin Nutr 1992; 55: 597S–601S.

36. Charuzi I, Ovnat A, Peiser J, et al. The effect of surgical weight reduction on sleep quality in obesity-related sleep apnea syndrome. Surgery 1985; 97: 535–538.

37. Jones KB Jr, Allen TV, Manas KJ, McGuinty DP, Wilder WM, Wadsworth ED. Roux-en-Y gastric bypass: an effective anti-reflux procedure. Obes Surg 1991; 1: 295–298.

38. Smith SC, Edwards CB, Goodman GN. Symptomatic and clinical improvement in morbidly obese patients with gastro-esophageal reflux disease following Roux-en-Y gastric bypass. Obes Surg 1997; 7: 470–484.

39. Sugerman HJ, Felton WL, Sismanis A, Salvant JB, Kellum JM. Effects of surgically induced weight loss on pseudotumor cerebri in morbid obesity. Neurology 1995; 45: 1655–1659.

40. Foley EF, Benotti PN, Borlase BC, Hollingshead J, Blackburn GL. Impact of gastric restrictive surgery on hypertension in the morbidly obese. Am J Surg 1992; 163: 294–297.

41. Carson JL, Ruddy ME, Duff AE, Holmes NJ, Cody RP, Brolin RE. The effect of gastric bypass surgery on hypertension in morbidly obese patients. Ann Int Med 1994; 154: 193–200.

42. Gleysteen JJ, Barboriak JJ, Sasse EA. Sustained coronary-risk-factor reduction after gastric bypass for morbid obesity. Am J Clin Nutr 1990; 51: 774–778.

43. Brolin RE, Kenler HA, Wilson AC, Kuo PT, Cody RP. Serum lipids after gastric bypass surgery for morbid obesity. Int J Obes 1990; 14: 939–950.

44. Alpert MA, Lambert CR, Terry BE, et al. Effect of weight loss on left ventricular mass in nonhypertensive morbidly obese patients. Am J Cardiol 1994; 73: 918–921.

45. Pories WJ, Swanson MS, MacDonald KG, Long SB, Morris PG, Brown BM, et al. Who would have thought it? An operation proves to be the most effective therapy for adult-onset diabetes mellitus? Ann Surg 1995; 222: 339–350.

46. Deitel M, Toan BT, Stone EM, Sutherland DJ, Wilk EJ. Sex hormone changes accompanying loss of massive excess weight. Gastroenterol Clin N Am 1987; 16: 511–516.
47. Bostman OM. Body mass index and height in patients requiring surgery for lumbar intervertebral disc herniation. Spine 1993; 18: 851–854.
48. Sugerman HJ, Sugerman EL, Wolfe L, Kellum JM, Schweitzer MA, DeMaria EJ. Risks–benefits of gastric bypass in morbidly obese patients with severe venous stasis disease. Gastroenterology 2000; 118: A1051.
49. Bump RC, Sugerman HJ, Fantl JA, et al. Obesity and lower urinary tract function in women: effects of surgically induced weight loss. Am J Obstet Gynecol 1992; 167: 392–397.
50. Stunkard AJ, Wadden TA. Psychological aspects of severe obesity. Am J Clin Nutr 1991; 55: 532S–534S.
51. Sugerman H, Windsor A, Bessos M, Kellum J, Reines H, DeMaria E. Effects of surgically induced weight loss on urinary bladder pressure, sagittal abdominal diameter and obesity co-morbidity. Int J Obes Relat Metab Disord 1998; 22: 230–235.
52. Karlsson J, Sjostrom L, Sullivan M. Swedish obese subjects (SOS): an intervention study of obesity. Two-year follow-up of health-related quality of life (HRQOL) and eating behavior after gastric surgery for severe obesity. Int J Obes Relat Metab Disord 1998; 22: 113–126.
53. Sjostrom CD, Lissner L, Sjostrom L. Relationships between changes in body composition and changes in cardiovascular risk factors: the SOS Intervention Study, Swedish Obese Subjects. Obes Res 1997; 5: 519–530.
54. Narbro K, Agren G, Jonsson E, Larsson B, Naslund I, Wedel H, Sjostrom L. Sick leave and disability pension before and after treatment for obesity: a report from the Swedish Obese Subjects (SOS) study. Int J Obes Relat Metab Disord 1999; 23: 619–624.
55. Sjostrom CD, Lissner L, Wedel H, Sjostrom L. Reduction in incidence of diabetes, hypertension and lipid disturbances after intentional weight loss included by bariatric surgery: the SOS Intervention Study. Obes Res 1999; 7: 477–484.
56. MacDonald KG Jr, Long SD, Swanson MS, Brown BM, Morris P, Dohm GL, Pories WJ. The gastric bypass operation reduces the progression and mortality of non-insulin-dependent diabetes mellitus. J Gastrointest Surg 1997; 1: 213–220.

Chapter 7

Managing Obesity to Lower the Risk of Cardiovascular Disease and Other Chronic Conditions

Kathleen J. Melanson, James B. Meigs, Kyle J. McInnis, and James M. Rippe

Obesity and overweight are chronic conditions affecting over half of the adult population in the United States, or an estimated 97 million individuals, resulting in serious health consequences (1–3). The escalating prevalence of obesity has occurred in both genders, virtually all ages, ethnic and socioeconomic groups (1,4) and in every region of the United States (5,6). This epidemic manifests serious impacts through various effects on morbidity and mortality, as well as through influences on quality of life and economic factors (3,4). Over 65% of individuals with a body mass index (BMI) of >27 kg/m² have at least one obesity-related comorbid condition (7). Some of these conditions are listed in Table 7-1. Classification criteria from the National Institutes of Health (NIH) and World Health Organization (WHO) for overweight and obesity according to BMI, as described in Chapter 1, are based on relative risk of morbidity and mortality (4). The prevalence of various comorbidities across classes of obesity and overweight for both genders, as indicated by cross-sectional data from National Health and Nutrition Evaluation Survey (NHANES) III, are listed in Table 7-2 (3). A lifestyle combining excessive energy intake

Table 7-1 Common Comorbidities of Obesity

Cardiovascular diseases	Sleep apnea
Impaired glucose tolerance	Gall bladder disease
Hyperinsulinemia	Osteoarthritis
Dyslipidemia	Some cancers
Type 2 diabetes mellitus	Reduced fertility
Hypertension	Polycystic ovarian disease
Stress incontinence	Non-alcoholic steatohepatitis
Hyperuricemia	Gout

and sedentary behavior has been cited as the second leading preventable cause of death in the United States, behind only smoking (8), and this trend is likely to worsen if the epidemic continues at its current pace (6).

This chapter examines the scientific evidence relating overweight and obesity to morbidity and mortality. Special attention is devoted to cardiovascular disease (CVD) and associated risk factors, because CVD is the leading cause of death in the United States, especially among obese individuals (4,9–11). The roles of weight gain and weight reduction in these relationships is also discussed. The final sections translate and apply existing research into the clinical arena of treatment and management of excess weight according to national and international guidelines.

OVERWEIGHT, OBESITY AND ALL-CAUSE MORTALITY

Based on data from five prospective cohort studies, an estimated 325,000 deaths can be attributed to obesity annually in Americans who have never smoked (11). This same analysis revealed that over 80% of deaths associated with conditions related to adiposity occur in individuals who have a BMI $> 30 \, kg/m^2$ (11). While the relationship between body weight and all cause mortality has been discussed for many years, some controversy still exists concerning this relationship, particularly at BMI $< 23 \, kg/m^2$. Some investigations have suggested that a J-shaped relationship exists between

Table 7-2 Prevalence of Comorbidity by Obesity Class and Sex. From Must et al (3) with permission.

Health Condition	Weight Status Category*					
	Underweight	Normal	Overweight	Obesity Class 1	Obesity Class 2	Obesity Class 3
Men (n = 6987)						
Type 2 diabetes mellitus	4.69	2.03	4.93	10.1	12.3	10.65
Gall bladder disease	6.96	1.93	3.39	5.38	5.8	10.17
Coronary heart disease	12.45	8.84	9.6	16.01	10.21	13.97
High blood cholesterol level	6.66	26.63	35.68	39.17	34.01	35.63
High blood pressure	23.38	23.47	34.16	48.95	65.48	64.53
Osteoarthritis	0.39	2.59	4.55	4.66	5.46	10.04
Women (n = 7689)						
Type 2 diabetes mellitus	4.76	2.38	7.12	7.24	13.16	19.89
Gall bladder disease	6.42	6.29	11.84	15.99	19.15	23.45
Coronary heart disease	12.07	6.87	11.13	12.56	12.31	19.22
High blood cholesterol level	13.36	26.89	45.59	40.37	40.96	36.39
High blood pressure	19.81	23.26	38.77	47.95	54.51	63.16
Osteoarthritis	7.79	5.22	8.51	9.94	10.39	17.19

* Estimates are weighted to account for the sample design. All data are percentages. Weight categories are based on the National Heart, Lung, and Blood Institute Classification. BMI, body mass index.

BMI and relative risk of death, because individuals with a BMI < 21 and >30 kg/m^2 exhibit increased relative risk of death compared to individuals with a BMI between 21 and 25 kg/m^2. For example, data from the Seven Countries Study in European men suggest that increased mortality is associated with BMI levels <18.5 kg/m^2 and >30.0 kg/m^2 (12). However, reverse causation may be playing a part in many reported findings, because much of the excess mortality associated with low BMI may be related to either pre-existing disease, current or former smoking, and/or alcoholism (13,14). Accounting for smoking and disease history explains much of the relationship between BMI and all-cause mortality, but increased risk remains apparent in all groups starting with BMI >26–30 kg/m^2 (13), as shown in Figure 7-1. Heavier men and women of all age groups have been shown to have higher mortality rates, even after accounting for smoking and concurrent comorbidities (13,15).

Increasing all-cause mortality with increasing severity of obesity has been reported from large-scale population studies of women (15) and men (16). However, the influence of body composition, rather than BMI alone, is gaining recognition in this relationship. In the latter study, in which body composition was assessed by total body potassium in 735 men, it was suggested that both low fat-free mass and high fat mass are predictive of mortality, creating a curve that is influenced by both ascending and descending functions. This compound function revealed that there was no lower limit of fat mass measured at which mortality increased, but men in the lowest quintile of fat-free mass exhibited significantly elevated mortality. High fat mass was associated with a 40% increase in total mortality (16). These, and other authors have proposed that such compounding of positive and negative linear effects on mortality from fat and fat-free mass, respectively, may at least partly explain J- or U-shaped relationships between BMI and mortality (17). The rationale for considering body composition in the relationship between BMI and mortality is strengthened by findings from a combined analysis of results from the Tecumseh and Framingham studies (18). In moderately obese

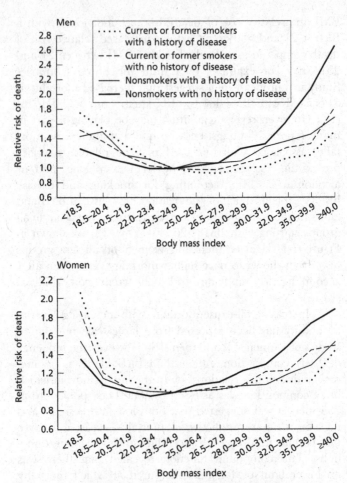

Figure 7-1 Relationship between body mass index and multivariate risk of all-cause mortality in men and women. (From Calle et al (13) with permission.)

individuals, overall weight loss was associated with increased mortality rates, but fat loss was associated with decreased mortality rates (18).

It has also been hypothesized that obesity is simply a marker for unhealthy lifestyle behaviors, such as physical inactivity and improper dietary habits, and that these factors, rather than obesity *per se*, may be exerting effects on morbidity and mortality (19). For example, lower cardiovascular mortality has been reported in men who have higher cardiorespiratory fitness levels compared to their unfit counterparts, independent of BMI (20,21). Many dietary factors, including total and saturated fat intake, as well as fruits, vegetables, and whole grains have also been implicated as modifiers of morbidity and mortality, especially from two of the leading causes of obesity-associated death in the United States: cardiovascular diseases (22) and cancers (23,24). Such lifestyle factors may be functioning independently or interactively in the relationship between body weight and mortality. Age has also been implicated as having an impact on this relationship (25). Methodological issues surrounding this area of research have been reviewed in detail elsewhere (14).

Weight change also influences obesity-related outcomes. Adult weight gains have been associated with increased mortality (15,26,27), and intentional weight losses with decreased mortality in some, but not all studies (26,28–31). Women in the Nurses' Health Study who gained >10 kg from age 18 years had significantly increased middle-aged cardiovascular, cancer and all-cause mortality compared to weight-stable women (15). In women with comorbidities related to obesity, intentional weight loss of any amount has been associated with significantly reduced all-cause mortality as well as mortality as a result of obesity-related cancers and diabetes (32). It has been postulated that the impact of intentional weight loss on reducing mortality may be dependent, at least in part, upon initial BMI and comorbidities (10,32), but this question is currently unresolved.

OVERWEIGHT, OBESITY AND CARDIOVASCULAR DISEASE RISK

Numerous epidemiological studies have shown that excess adiposity as assessed by BMI is a major risk factor for various chronic diseases, including CVD particularly coronary heart disease (CHD), as well as hypertension, dyslipidemia, and type 2 diabetes (8,33–35). In a prospective study of over 1 million men and women, obesity was most predictive of CVD death compared to other causes of mortality, especially in men (13). Risks for all-cause mortality, CVD deaths, and other chronic conditions were significantly elevated for women with BMI >25 kg/m^2, and for men with BMI >26.5 kg/m^2 (13). In a study of 25,000 nurses, those with a BMI >32 kg/m^2 had four times the risk of death from·CVD compared with those who had a BMI < 19 kg/m^2, and adult weight gain of ≥ 10 kg was predictive of all-cause, CVD, and cancer death (15).

Coronary Heart Disease

The American Heart Association (AHA) has identified obesity as a major modifiable risk factor for CHD, imparting similar cardiovascular risk as hypertension, hyperlipidemia, smoking, and sedentary lifestyle (9). Major population-based studies including the Framingham Heart Study (36,37), the Nurses' Health Study (15), and the Health Professionals Follow-up Study (38) have all shown that obesity represents a significant risk factor for CHD, independent of other well-established CHD risk factors.

In both the Health Professionals Follow-up (38) and the Nurses' Health Study (15), elevated BMI was strongly associated with increased risk of CHD after controlling for several other risk factors. In these analyses, data on blood pressure or plasma lipids were unavailable, therefore resulting in possible incomplete control of confounders. Nevertheless, even overweight individuals (BMI 25–28.9 kg/m^2) exhibited significantly elevated relative risk (72% in middle-aged men) for CHD. Progressive increases in CHD risk have been reported for men and women across all BMI categories (15,38). The relationship between relative body weight and risk for fatal or non-fatal CHD may be modified by subject characteristics such as gender, age, fitness level, ethnicity, and body fat distribution (9,15,20,37,39).

Stroke

Data from the Nurses' Health Study have shown that obese women have a significantly increased risk of ischemic and total (but not hemorrhagic) stroke (40). Compared to women with a BMI of $<21\,kg/m^2$, women with a BMI of $27-28.9\,kg/m^2$ had a relative risk of stroke of 1.75. Women with a BMI of $29-31.9\,kg/m^2$ had a relative risk of 1.90, and those with a BMI of $32\,kg/m^2$ or more had a relative risk of 2.37 of ischemic or total stroke. In addition, weight gains $>11\,kg$ during adult years significantly increased the risk of ischemic and total stroke in the Nurses' Health Study (40). Visceral adiposity may also increase risk of stroke. Longitudinal data in men have shown tertiles of abdominal adiposity to be progressively linked to stroke, independent of BMI (41). In a 14.8-year prospective study in 7735 British males, the age-adjusted risk for all types of stroke increased beyond BMI of $22\,kg/m^2$, but after adjustment for other lifestyle factors this trend became non-significant ($P = 0.06$) (42).

Left Ventricular Dysfunction/Congestive Heart Failure

With increased body mass comes increased stroke volume, cardiac output, peripheral resistance, and diastolic dysfunction, resulting in elevated blood pressure and enlarged left ventricular mass. In severe obesity, dilatated cardiomyopathy may predispose to arrhythmias (10). As a result of these direct effects on the heart, obesity has been identified as a cardiovascular risk factor beyond risks imparted through CHD in particular (43).

According to data from the 26-year follow-up of over 5000 Framingham Heart Study participants, risk for congestive heart failure (CHF) increased by a factor of 2.5–3.0 comparing leanest to heaviest subjects (36). This was observed in both genders, independent of age, total cholesterol level, systolic blood pressure, cigarette smoking, type 2 diabetes, or left ventricular hypertrophy (36). It has been hypothesized that the effects of obesity on CHF may be related to hypertension and left ventricular hypertrophy. However, abnormalities of both left ventricular mass and function may be seen in obese individuals even in the absence of hypertension.

OVERWEIGHT, OBESITY AND CARDIOVASCULAR RISK FACTORS

Hypertension

The risk of hypertension increases two- to fourfold with increasing body weight (44). Obesity is the single strongest predictor of blood pressure, associated with an estimated 40–70% of cases of hypertension in the United States (9,44). The AHA has stated that hypertension can be directly attributed to obesity in most patients (43) and that obesity predicts coronary atherosclerosis, independent of several other established risk factors (9).

A significant relationship between obesity and hypertension, independent of age, smoking, alcohol consumption, and electrolyte excretion was reported in the Intersalt study (45). A variety of mechanisms have been postulated to explain the links between obesity and hypertension (46). Elevated cardiac output, increased peripheral resistance and reduced venous compliance have all been observed in obese individuals (46). In addition, insulin resistance and hyperinsulinemia, which often accompany obesity, increase sympathetic tone and renal sodium retention, further contributing to increased risk of hypertension in obese individuals (44).

In a study of hypertensive and normotensive obese patients, weight losses of 10.4 kg were accompanied by reductions of 10.3 mmHg systolic and 8.0 mmHg diastolic blood pressure (47). Another trial of moderately obese hypertensive individuals reported systolic blood pressure to be reduced by 0.43 mmHg per kg of weight loss, and diastolic blood pressure by 0.33 mmHg per kg weight loss (48). Weight loss in hypertensive patients also reduces concomitant cardiovascular risk factors such as diabetes and dyslipidemia (49).

The Trials of Hypertension Prevention (TOHP I and II) which studied over 2000 borderline hypertensive patients demonstrated that weight loss was more effective than sodium restriction, stress management, or supplementation with calcium, magnesium, potassium, or fish oil for blood pressure reduction (48,50,51). In TOHP I, weight losses of 5.7 kg at 6 months were associated with significant reductions in systolic and diastolic blood pressure. By 18 months some weight regain was observed, such that body weights were only 3.9 kg below initial weights, but blood pressure was still significantly reduced below original levels (systolic: −2.9 mmHg; diastolic: −2.3 mmHg). When the entire group of volunteers was divided into quintiles of weight change, it was observed that patients who lost the most weight achieved the greatest declines in both systolic and diastolic blood pressure. This trend was seen at 6, 12, and 18 months (48). In TOHP II, body weights of patients followed until 36 months were shown to be 2.2 kg below original weights in the intervention group, as compared to a 2.2-kg weight gain in the control group (51). At this point, both systolic and diastolic blood pressures were significantly reduced in the weight loss groups below their starting levels, as well as compared to the control group.

The Swedish Obese Subjects (SOS) intervention study examined the relationship between changes in body composition over 2 years and changes in cardiovascular risk factors in 842 men and women treated for obesity by surgery or standard intervention. As shown in Figure 7-2, adjusted blood pressure decreases were apparent with increasing weight loss, and were observable after a loss of 5–10 kg. Individuals who gained weight during this study showed trends of increased systolic and diastolic blood pressure (52).

Weight gains are associated with increases in blood pressure (53,54) and weight reduction has been associated with decreases in blood pressure (54), independent of sodium restriction (55,56). Weight reduction of as little as 10 lb (4.5 kg) reduces blood pressure in a large proportion of hypertensive overweight persons, enhances effectiveness of antihypertensive agents, reduces concomitant cardiovascular risk factors, and may improve compliance to pharmacotherapy (4,49).

Although the mechanistic relationships between altered body weight and changes in blood pressure are not

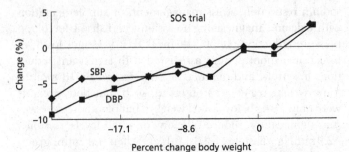

Figure 7-2 Change in blood pressure in the Swedish Obese Subjects (SOS) trial with sustained weight loss of 5–10 kg. SBP, systolic blood pressure; DBP, diastolic blood pressure. (From Sjöström et al (52) with permission.)

completely clarified, several possible mechanisms have been postulated, and may vary in the degree to which they play a part in different individuals (57–60). Examples include changes in extracellular volume and thus cardiac output, sympathetic nervous system activity, peripheral vascular resistance, insulin resistance, aberrations in the renin–angiotensin–aldosterone system and, in severe obesity, direct effects on the heart (61). Based on sound evidence on the relationship between obesity and hypertension, two expert committees have recommended that weight loss should be attempted in obese hypertensive patients, for 3–6 months in stage 1 hypertension before taking a pharmacologic approach (4,49). Weight reduction, even at modest levels, has been implicated as the most effective non-pharmacologic treatment of hypertension in obese patients (62).

Dyslipidemias
Multiple lipid abnormalities are associated with obesity (63–65), typified by atherogenic dyslipidemia that includes elevated triglycerides, low high-density lipoprotein (HDL) levels, high low-density lipoprotein (LDL) levels and increased concentrations of small dense LDL particles (39). Small dense LDL particles are commonly associated with the obese state, and are particularly atherogenic because of

their susceptibility to oxidation (39). Depressed HDL cholesterol, and elevated levels of triglycerides, total cholesterol, and LDL cholesterol have all been related to higher BMI in men and women (35,39). According to data from NHANES III, BMI is significantly associated with abnormal plasma lipids, as well as hypertension, after controlling for age, race, ethnicity, education, and smoking (35).

In the PROCAM study, a linear relationship was observed between BMI and the prevalence of elevated cholesterol levels in 20–29-year-old individuals; 53% of those with BMI >30 kg/m^2 had elevated cholesterol levels (66). For individuals in the age range of 50–59 years, elevated cholesterol levels were apparent in 71–77% of the individuals studied, regardless of BMI. Similar trends were reported for LDL cholesterol, but high triglycerides and low HDL were more prevalent in more obese quartiles, regardless of age (66).

A meta-analysis examining 70 trials of dietary weight loss revealed significant decreases in total cholesterol, LDL cholesterol, and triglycerides in individuals with dyslipidemia (67). Significant improvements in HDL cholesterol were achieved in individuals with reduced stabilized weight (67). In the SOS study, weight losses of 5–40 kg were associated with decreased total cholesterol and increased HDL. Both of these improvements in plasma lipid profiles were stronger with greater losses (52). A number of studies have demonstrated that clinically relevant changes in cholesterol and HDL ratios can occur with weight loss as little as 5–10% of initial body weight (4). Modest weight losses (5–9%) sustained over 2 years in men and women have been shown to produce significant reductions in plasma concentrations of triglycerides, glucose, and insulin, as well as blood pressure (68).

Guidelines from the National Cholesterol Education Program (1993) state that diet therapy is a vital component of lowering blood lipid levels and, in overweight patients, weight reduction must be an integral part of dietary therapy. In obese individuals, the AHA Step I and II diets have been shown to reduce plasma triglycerides, total cholesterol, and LDL cholesterol, although HDL cholesterol may also decline

(69). Nevertheless, when these diets include weight loss, further significant reductions in plasma triglycerides, total cholesterol, and LDL cholesterol result, but plasma HDL often increases, thus resulting in overall improvements in plasma lipid profile (70). These improvements are further enhanced by the inclusion of physical activity (70). In a study comparing obese individuals consuming an AHA diet over 9 months with or without weight loss, significant improvements in lipoprotein lipids (including increased HDL cholesterol) were observed in the group that lost weight over time, as compared to their weight-maintaining counterparts (71). Similar results have been reported in numerous studies of varying design, as described in depth in a recent meta-analysis (70). Favorable changes in plasma lipid profiles correlate strongly with weight reduction (52), which is the basis for weight reduction recommendations in obese dyslipidemic individuals (4).

Type 2 Diabetes

Hyperinsulinemia, hyperglycemia, and insulin resistance are positively correlated with BMI and visceral adiposity (33,39,72), as are glucose intolerance and type 2 diabetes mellitus (10,72,73). Approximately 85–90% of all Americans with type 2 diabetes are obese (33). The increased risk of type 2 diabetes escalates dramatically across classes of overweight and obesity. In the US Male Health Professionals Study, men with a BMI of 25–26.9 kg/m^2 had 2.2 times the risk of developing type 2 diabetes compared with men with a BMI < 23 kg/m^2. In males with a BMI > 35 kg/m^2 the risk of developing type 2 diabetes was 42 times that of a man whose BMI was < 23 kg/m^2 (74). In the Nurses' Health Study, women who had a BMI of 24–24.9 kg/m^2 had five times the risk of developing type 2 diabetes compared to women with a BMI < 22 kg/m^2. In women with a BMI ≥ 31 kg/m^2, risk of developing diabetes was 40 times greater than women with a BMI < 22 kg/m^2 (72).

In addition to the effects of obesity itself, both of these studies demonstrated that significant weight gains (>10 kg) during adult years were significant determinants of the risk for developing type 2 diabetes (72,74). Obesity and excess visceral adipose accumulation promote insulin resistance and compensatory hyperinsulinemia, leading to impaired glucose tolerance and eventually type 2 diabetes. Increased adult weight gain is associated with increased relative risk for clinical diabetes, and this effect has been shown to be more apparent in individuals with an elevated BMI at age 18 years (72). The prevalence of hyperinsulinemia, insulin resistance, and insulin hypersecretion has been shown to be positively correlated with BMI (4,10,33,75,76).

Weight reduction consistently results in a variety of health benefits related to glucose intolerance in obese individuals (33). In diabetic patients at various stages of disease progression, weight loss proves to be highly effective in improving insulin sensitivity and glycemic control (33,77–80). Normalization of carbohydrate metabolism has been reported in 141 of 163 morbidly obese diabetic patients who had undergone gastric bypass surgery and maintained weight loss over 10 years (81). Additionally, weight loss reliably produces improved lipid profiles in obese diabetic patients (82).

Recent data from the Framingham Study have demonstrated that sustained modest weight losses of only 1–2 kg/year over 16 years in obese men and women protected against the development of diabetes (83). Compared to weight-stable obese subjects, risk reduction in individuals maintaining weight loss during this time ranged from 37 to 66%, depending on initial BMI. With weight regain, the risk of developing diabetes was 30% as compared to weight stability.

The amount of weight loss required to produce clinical improvements in type 2 diabetes remains somewhat controversial. Some studies have suggested that significant improvements in glycemic control may occur with 5–9% weight loss (82), while others have required more than 10% weight loss (78–80). Varying data from such studies may have resulted from differences in dietary practices, variability in subject characteristics, and the nature and timing of the measurements.

Treatment strategies involving diet and exercise work at the levels of the skeletal muscle and adipose to directly decrease insulin resistance (33,75). Weight loss may function in diabetes by reducing hepatic glucose output and improving insulin sensitivity both through the decline in adipose tissue mass as well as through a direct effect of the hypocaloric state itself (33,84).

Hemostasis

Obesity, particularly abdominal obesity, is associated with hemostatic risk factors for CVD, including increased fibrinogen and plasminogen activator inhibitor-1 (PAI-1) levels (85). Fibrinogen levels have been shown to correlate with BMI, waist circumference, and plasma insulin, and the degree of weight loss is predictive of reductions in plasma fibrinogen levels (86). Positive trends have been reported across quintiles of fasting insulin levels for BMI, PAI-1 antigen, fibrinogen, and plasma lipids (with a negative trend for HDL-cholesterol), suggesting a relationship between hyperinsulinemia and impaired fibrinolytic potential (76).

Modest weight losses have been shown to improve hemostatic risk factors in men and women (86,87), and weight gain has been shown to significantly worsen these factors (86). In a study examining weight reduction of 13.6 kg followed by weight maintenance, sustained decreases in plasma fibrinogen and PAI-1 antigen were observed in addition to decreases in total cholesterol and triglycerides and increases in HDL cholesterol, regardless of the weight loss strategy undertaken (88). One may hypothesize that impaired fibrinolysis accounts for residual effects in the relationship between adiposity and CVD after controlling for standard CVD risk factors. No study has examined this possibility to date.

Risk Factor Clustering

Data from NHANES III show that obese individuals have a 65% chance of having at least one additional risk factor for CHD, such as hypertension, dyslipidemia, or type 2 diabetes (89). In the Framingham Heart Study, obese men and women had a 48 and 54% chance, respectively, of having at least two other metabolic risk factors for heart disease (7).

Obesity was associated with excessive presence of all major risk factors except cigarette smoking. This clustering of risk factors has serious consequences, because relative risk of CHD increases linearly with increasing number of risk factors in a given individual (89). In the United States, 55% of all heart disease in men and 78% of all heart disease in women occurs in individuals with two or more cardiovascular risk factors (7). Individuals with two or more risk factors for heart disease suffer over half of all heart disease worldwide (90).

More than 12,000 NHANES I participants who did not have CHD during the study were followed-up to examine multiple risk factors, including hypertension, hypercholesterolemia, weight gain, smoking, and type 2 diabetes (89). In younger patients, the presence of even one risk factor more than doubled the incidence of CHD. Patients with four or five risk factors had an eightfold risk of CHD. Even in older patients, there was a linear relationship between the number of risk factors and incidence of CHD.

Most individuals at risk for CVD or type 2 diabetes have multiple risk factors for comorbid conditions (91). Obesity and weight gain are important determinants of risk factor clustering because several hemodynamic and metabolic abnormalities tend to cluster together in obese individuals (76,91). Mild abnormalities in hypertension, hyperinsulinemia, and dyslipidemia can act synergistically to increase the risk of CHD (91). Obesity has been postulated as an underlying cause of risk factor clustering because atherogenic risk factor clustering worsens with increased weight (91), although it is also plausible that risk factor clustering in obesity may be the cause of CVD. This issue of co-occurrence of CVD risk factors in obesity, and the direction of causality, must be systematically investigated in further detail.

Visceral Adiposity

Many studies have shown that abdominal obesity imparts additional risk of CHD and ischemic heart disease above that exerted by an elevated BMI alone (39,92,93). Visceral adiposity has significantly predicted CHD mortality in epidemiologic studies of men (74), and women (15).

In the Iowa Women's Health Study, central adiposity conferred additional CHD risk in every tertile of BMI (92). In NHANES I, central obesity correlated with an increased relative risk of CHD of 1.62 in women and 1.56 in men (93). Elevated waist:hip ratio (WHR) was also a strong predictor of CHD mortality in the US Male Health Professional Study (74), a study of US Army Veterans (94), and the Nurses' Health Study (15). An independent relationship has also been demonstrated between visceral adiposity and ischemic heart disease (95). Obese individuals with high levels of visceral adiposity tend to have elevated plasma triglycerides, increased formation of dense LDL particles and low HDL levels (96–99) as compared to obese individuals with low levels of visceral adiposity. However, regardless of the distribution of excess adiposity, obese individuals consistently have higher triglycerides and lower HDL as compared to non-obese individuals (65), as depicted in Figure 7-3.

Aberrations in glucose metabolism are also a representative feature of the insulin-resistance syndrome (or "Syndrome X") that is prevalent in individuals with abdominal obesity (79). Visceral adiposity represents a risk factor for insulin resistance that is independent of BMI (65). The associated hyperinsulinemia, interactions between glucose and lipid metabolism, and the lipolytic nature of visceral adipocytes are factors that contribute to the adverse changes in plasma lipid profiles accompanying the accumulation of central body fat. Exaggerated areas under glucose and insulin response curves have been observed in obese males and females with high levels of visceral fat compared to their counterparts with low levels of visceral fat (100). Excess central adiposity, expressed as WHR, has repeatedly been demonstrated as a risk factor for type 2 diabetes in men. The probability of developing type 2 diabetes over 13.5 years in relation to tertiles of initial BMI and WHR has been shown to increase linearly (75). While there is a continuum of risk associated with increased waist circumference, current

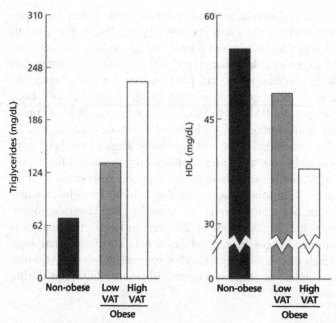

VAT = visceral adipose tissue = visceral fat

Figure 7-3 Visceral fat levels, plasma triglycerides and high-density lipoprotein in non-obese and obese women. (From Després (65) with permission.)

guidelines from the National Heart, Lung and Blood Institute (NHLBI) and WHO categorize abdominal adiposity, denoting waist circumferences >35 inches in women and >40 inches in men as the highest risk categories (4) (see Tables 1-1a and 1-1b, Chapter 1).

Weight reduction in viscerally obese individuals reduces plasma triglyceride levels to a greater extent than in individuals with more peripheral adiposity (101). In the SOS study, changes in multiple CVD risk factors were followed over 2 years in obese individuals whose body weight changes ranged from −95.5 to +30.6 kg, and body composition was assessed by computed tomography (52). Reductions in both subcutaneous and visceral adipose were associated with improvements in risk factors, and the opposite held true for gains in these adipose depots. For women, changes in body weight were the single best predictor of changes in risk factor status, whereas in men, changes in waist circumference and BMI had similar roles. Nevertheless, in both genders, modest weight reductions of about 10 kg (from BMI 32 to 29 kg/m^2) have been shown to result in significant reductions in visceral adipose content (97). To date, no specific diet and exercise strategies have been conclusively proven to preferentially reduce visceral fat depots (102), but because these depots are more responsive to treatment than subcutaneous adipose, standard weight management strategies should be effective for viscerally obese patients (39). A review of 23 intervention studies that measured changes in visceral fat depots concluded that high levels of overall body fat and of visceral fat were the two best predictors of selective visceral adipose mobilization during weight loss (103).

Weight Gain

In addition to obesity and visceral adiposity, adult weight gain itself has been associated with increased risk factors for CHD, and significantly predictive of CHD events (74). Compared with women of stable weight (±0.5 kg), the relative risk of CHD ranges from 1.25 in women who gain 5–7.9 kg as an adult, to 2.65 for women who gain 20 kg or more (15). The relative risk for hypertension has been positively correlated with adult weight gain in multivariate analyses (44,54). Modest adult weight gains of 5–10 kg lead to a relative risk of 1.5 and weight gains of 25 kg impart a relative risk of almost 7 as compared to weight stability. Considerable weight gain in men after the age of 21 also correlates significantly with increased risk of CHD, type 2 diabetes, hypertension, and stroke (74). Data from women in the Cancer Prevention Study I revealed that both obesity and adult weight gain were determinants of CHD risk (32). The combination of these newly emerging data underscores the importance of preventing weight gain as well as addressing established obesity.

Degree of Weight Loss and Cardiovascular Disease Risk Factor Reduction

The degree of weight loss required to yield significant reduction in risk factors for CHD is often relatively modest. Weight losses of 5–10% in obese individuals with type 2 diabetes, hypertension, or dyslipidemia have resulted in improved glycemic control, reduced blood pressure, and improved lipid profiles (4,80,104). Normalization of metabolic risk factors has been reported for women and men who lost on average 8 and 14 kg, respectively, over 15 weeks, yet were still clinically obese. Such risk factors included plasma insulin, total cholesterol, LDL cholesterol, HDL cholesterol, triglycerides, and glucose tolerance (105). Morbidly obese men and women treated surgically for obesity and followed for 5–7 years exhibited significant sustained improvements in multiple coronary risk factors, including plasma HDL: total cholesterol ratio, hypertension, and diabetes (106). The benefits of modest weight loss on multiple risk factors and outcomes provide impetus for encouraging even moderate weight reduction in obese patients, especially those with comorbidities. This serves as the basis for the recommendations from the NIH for an initial weight loss goal of 10% of body weight (4).

The importance of modest weight losses in reducing multiple risk factors has received much attention, but the necessity of maintaining such weight loss needs greater emphasis. Recent data have suggested that weight reductions >10% must be sustained in order to keep some cardiovascular risk factors in their improved state (107). Reversal of improvements in some risk factors has been associated with weight regain. In a 2-year study of 25 women who had undergone a 20% weight reduction over 48 weeks, those women who maintained a weight loss of at least 10% still exhibited improvements in plasma lipids, whereas those who maintained a loss of only 5–10% of their initial weight showed no significant improvements in plasma lipids compared to prediet baseline (107). Differences were also apparent among groups; the greater the percentage weight loss maintained, the greater the reductions in total and LDL cholesterol. Similar findings of reversal of improvements in some risk factors with partial recidivism after weight loss have also been reported in other studies (52,108,109).

A 4-year study after weight reduction in women found that the amount of weight regained was correlated with increases in blood pressure, triglycerides, and cholesterol and decreases in HDL (110). Women who chose to exercise regularly during the follow-up regained less weight than those who did not, which may partly explain improvements in blood pressure and plasma lipids (70). It has been hypothesized that some of the reported risk factor reductions with moderate weight loss may be directly related to the hypocaloric state (107), and that the degree of weight loss and maintenance required for clinical improvements may depend upon initial BMI (52,107). Further research is required in larger numbers of individuals to determine the levels of weight reduction that must be maintained over the long term in order to retain the improvements in risk factors achieved through weight loss itself.

OVERWEIGHT, OBESITY AND OTHER COMORBID CONDITIONS

Cancers

Certain forms of cancer, particularly colon, prostate, endometrial, and postmenopausal but not premenopausal breast cancer, have been associated with elevated BMI. However, in many studies, the confounding influences from body weight and other factors such as dietary composition and lifestyle behaviors are difficult to discern (23,104). In a 12-year longitudinal study of 750,000 adults, cancer mortality ratios were 1.55 for obese men and 1.33 for obese women (111). The types of cancers affecting obese men most frequently were colorectal and prostate, whereas obese women suffered from most endometrial, gall bladder, cervical, ovarian, and breast cancers (111). The relationship between body weight and colon cancer appears to be stronger in men than women (23,111). A BMI >29 kg/m² has been associated with half of the cases of both endometrial and breast cancers in postmenopausal women (112). In the Nurses' Health Study, elevated cancer mortality was found in obese women (15), and adult weight gain was associated with increased risk of breast cancer, independent of BMI (113). In the Cancer Prevention Study I, women with obesity-related health conditions intentionally losing any amount of body weight exhibited a 40–50% reduction in cancer mortality, but this relationship was not observed in obese women with no pre-existing comorbidities (32). The relationship between weight reduction and cancer risk warrants further investigation.

Osteoarthritis

Cross-sectional data from NHANES III showed progressive increases in the prevalence of osteoarthritis across all classes of overweight and obesity in adults, particularly women (3) (Table 7-2). Other population studies have supported these findings (114,115). Weight-bearing joints, especially the knees, and to a lesser extent the hips, are the most commonly affected by osteoarthritis in obese patients, although joints in the hands are also frequently affected (116). The development of obesity-related osteoarthritis most likely occurs through increased mechanical stress on the joints, although systemic factors may also be involved (116–118). It has been estimated that for every 5 kg of weight gain, the risk of knee arthritis increases by 35% (119). In the Framingham Study, weight losses of approximately 5.1 kg over 10 years were associated with over 50% reduction in the odds ratio for developing osteoarthritis (120). However, more data are required to discern the effectiveness of various weight management approaches in reducing osteoarthritis in obese patients (116).

Sleep Apnea

In both men and women, the incidence of sleep apnea increases with excess body weight, particularly BMI > 30 kg/m² (121–123). Sleep apnea is characterized by loud snoring and cessation of breathing for at least 10 s, often followed by a brief awakening. Excess weight from adipose tissue on the chest wall and abdomen decreases compliance of respiratory function and reduces lung volume, eventually leading to hypoventilation (124). In addition to causing daytime fatigue, sleep apnea can lead to arterial hypoxemia, pulmonary and systemic hypertension, cardiac arrythmias and, in severe cases, can be fatal (4,10,124). Weight reduction has been associated with improvements in symptoms of sleep apnea (4,124–126) and weight regains associated with return of symptoms (125).

Gall Bladder Diseases

As shown in Table 7-2, NHANES III data indicate that gall bladder disease prevalence increases across all categories of overweight and obesity (3). However, this association is modified by gender and age. In males below age 55 years, body weight imparts a stronger risk for gall bladder diseases, whereas the gradient is not as strong in older men. Women, who experience twice the prevalence of this condition compared to men, show steady increases in gall bladder diseases with excess body weight, regardless of age (3). Central adiposity has also been implicated in risk for gallstones in men (127). Longitudinal data corroborate this relationship between gall bladder diseases and body weight, especially in severe obesity (128,129). Increased biliary cholesterol and altered gall bladder motility have been implicated in the etiology of obesity-induced gall bladder diseases (130). During negative energy balance, risk of gallstone formation may be increased because of increased lipid turnover, so caution should be practised in prescribing rapid weight loss to patients with or at risk for gall bladder diseases (129,130).

Liver Conditions

Hepatic and portal inflammation, fibrosis and fatty infiltration have been reported in obese individuals, particularly those with concomitant hyperinsulinemia and/or type 2 diabetes (130,131). These features, which may resemble those of alcoholic liver disease, but in the absence of excess alcohol intake, are referred to as non-alcoholic steatohepatitis (NASH) (10,131). It has been reported that 70–100% of NASH patients are 10–40% overweight (131,132), but that the condition can be reversed with weight loss (132). However, as with the risk of gall bladder diseases, rapid weight loss should be avoided in patients with or at risk for NASH, because the hypocaloric state may exacerbate the condition (10,130).

Weight Management and Risk Reduction

A vast literature supports the concept of treating the individual risk factors for CHD separately as a means of lowering CHD risk. Extensive research has shown that treatment of high blood pressure reduces the risk of both CHD and stroke (62). Numerous randomized prospective trials have shown that effective treatment of dyslipidemias (particularly total cholesterol reduction) leads to decreased risk of CHD (70). Thus, treating these individual risk factors for CHD in obese individuals is based on a large body of evidence demonstrating that effective control of these individual risk factors lowers the risk of CHD. The relationship between effective treatment of type 2 diabetes and lowering the risk of CHD is not as clearly demonstrated as the previous two risk factors. To date, there is no conclusive evidence that strategies to lower blood glucose result in decreased risk of CHD (33).

Despite decades of extensive research, much remains to be elucidated regarding the relationships among obesity, weight changes, and CVD, especially causal links. No direct evidence exists to prove that weight loss is directly responsible for decreases in CVD events, independent of associated reductions in other risk factors (10). However, the prevalence of obesity, and accumulating data associating adiposity with CHD risk, as well as possible interaction with other risk factors for CHD, emphasize the need for action and progress. Existing data, as discussed in this chapter, provide robust evidence that obesity therapy should be considered standard treatment to reduce the risk of CHD in obese patients. Treating obesity as first-line therapy may simultaneously reduce multiple risk factors for CHD and may ultimately reduce risk of CHD itself. This strategy seems particularly worthwhile given the recent understanding that multiple risk factors for CHD tend to cluster in obese individuals (91).

Less information is available on the long-term effects of weight loss on CHD itself rather than its risk factors. This has been largely attributed to the high incidence of recidivism in clinical weight loss trials. In the Cancer Prevention Study, a long-term follow-up study of over 750,000 women, those with obesity-related conditions such as diabetes and hypertension who underwent intentional weight loss experienced a 9% reduction in CHD mortality (32). Women with no pre-existing illness derived no benefit from intentional weight loss. In this cohort, intentional weight losses of up to 20 lb (9 kg) were associated with reductions in adjusted all-cause mortality of approximately 20%. These reductions were partially a result of reduced cancer- and diabetes-related mortality as well as reductions in CHD mortality. With such modest intentional weight losses, adjusted mortality rates from obesity-related cancers declined by approximately 50% (32).

Large-scale prospective trials are needed to resolve the issue of the effect of intentional weight loss on CHD mortality. In the meantime, the positive association of relatively modest weight loss to reduction in risk factors for CHD provides supportive evidence for the applicability of weight management as first-line therapy for obese individuals who have hypertension, type 2 diabetes, and dyslipidemias as a means of CHD risk reduction. These facts have been incorporated in nationally recognized evidence-based guidelines for the treatment of hypertension, dyslipidemias, and diabetes. The Joint National Committee (JNC) VI Guidelines for the treatment of hypertension in obese individuals list weight loss as first-line therapy (49). According to the guidelines established by the National Cholesterol Education Program, weight loss is first-line therapy for individuals with dyslipidemia who are overweight (133). According to guidelines established by the American Diabetes Association, weight loss represents first-line therapy for overweight and obese individuals with type 2 diabetes (134).

Viable strategies are becoming increasingly available for the successful treatment of obesity. For example, proper nutrition, regular physical activity, and behavior modification have all been demonstrated, under proper circumstances, to result in effective weight management (107,135,136). When appropriate, pharmacologic or surgical options may serve as adjuvant treatments. At present, the unfortunate reality is that successful maintenance of weight loss is rare (137). However, the advancement of research on various dimensions of weight management is providing increasing resources for overcoming barriers to weight loss (4). Furthermore, data from the National Weight Registry (NWR) continue to offer insight into how recidivism can be avoided (138,139), and hope for those who feel that maintenance of weight loss is insurmountable (140).

CONCLUSIONS

Abundant data support the existence of a strong and global relationship of obesity to all-cause mortality, CVD, and other comorbid conditions. Obesity is particularly associated with CHD risk, and is related to multiple risk factors for CHD including hypertension, type 2 diabetes, dyslipidemia, and impaired hemostasis. However, fewer data are currently available to describe direct causal relationships among obesity, weight changes, risk factors, and CVD events. Effective treatment of obesity, often with relatively modest reductions of 5–10% of initial body weight, decreases risk factors for CHD, but the resulting changes in risk for CVD morbidity and mortality remain to be elucidated. In addition to obesity, adult weight gain and abdominal distribution of excess adiposity have been reported as contributors to CHD. Although sufficient data are not yet available to elucidate the role of weight reduction in decreasing CVD events, national and international guidelines support obesity treatment as an important strategy for CHD risk factor reduction. The availability of data regarding risk reduction for other comorbidities of obesity varies with the condition but, in most cases, weight management is appropriate. Effective evidence-based clinical strategies for weight management are now available that are likely to improve the health and well-being of obese patients.

REFERENCES

1. Kuczmarski RJ, Flegal KM, Campbell SM, Johnson CL. Increasing prevalence of overweight among US adults: the National Health and Nutrition Examination Surveys 1960–1991. JAMA 1994; 272: 205–211.
2. World Health Organization. Obesity: preventing and managing the global epidemic. Report of a WHO Consultation presented at the World Health Organization, 3–5 June 1997; Geneva Switzerland. Publication WHO/NUT/NCD/98.1.
3. Must A, Spandano J, Coakley EH, Feild A, Colditz G, Dietz W. The disease burden associated with overweight and obesity. JAMA 1999; 282: 1523–1529.
4. National Institutes of Health. Clinical guidelines on the identification, evaluation, and treatment of overweight and obesity in adults: the evidence report. Bethesda, MD: National Heart, Lung and Blood Institute, June 1998.
5. Mokdad AH, Serdula MK, Dietz WH, Bowman BA, Marks JS, Koplan JP. The spread of the obesity epidemic in the United States, 1991–1998. JAMA 1999; 282: 1519–1522.
6. Mokdad AH, Serdula MK, Dietz WH, Bowman BA, Marks JS, Koplan JP. The continuing epidemic of obesity in the United States. JAMA 2000; 284: 1650–1651.
7. Wilson P, Kannel WB. Clustering of risk factors, obesity and Syndrome X. Nutr Clin Care 1998; 1: 44–50.
8. McGinnis JM, Foege WH. Actual causes of death in the United States. JAMA 1993; 270: 2207–2212.
9. Eckel R. Obesity and heart disease: A statement for the healthcare professionals from the Nutrition Committee, American Heart Association. Circulation 1997; 96: 3248–3250.
10. National Task Force on the Prevention and Treatment of Obesity. Arch Intern Med 2000; 160: 898–904.
11. Allison DB, Fontaine KR, Manson JE, Stevens J, VanItallie TB. Annual deaths attributable to obesity in the United States. JAMA 1999; 282: 1530–1538.
12. Visscher TLS, Seidell JC, Menotti A, Blackburn H, Nissinen A, Feskens EJM, Kromhout D. Underweight and overweight

in relation to mortality among men aged 40–59 and 50–69 years. Am J Epidemiol 2000; 151: 660–666.

13. Calle E, Thun MJ, Petrelli JM, Rodrigues C, Heath CW. Body mass index and mortality in a prospective cohort of US adults. N Engl J Med 1999; 34: 1097–1105.

14. Seidell JC, Visscher TLS, Hoogeveen RT. Overweight and obesity in the mortality rate data: current evidence and research issues. Med Sci Sports Exerc 1999; 31: S597–S601.

15. Manson JE, Willet WC, Stamfer MJ, Colditz GA, Hunter DJ, Hankinson SE, Hennekens CH, Speizer FE. Body weight and mortality among women. N Engl J Med 1995; 333: 677–685.

16. Heitmann BL, Erkison H, Ellsinger B-M, Mikkelsen KL, Larsson B. Mortality associated with body fat, fat-free mass and body mass index among 60-year-old Swedish men: a 22 year follow-up. The study of men born in 1913. Int J Obes 2000; 24: 33–37.

17. Allison DB, Faith MS, Heo M, Kotler DP. Hypothesis concerning the U-shaped relation between body mass index and mortality. Am J Epidemiol 1997; 146: 339–349.

18. Allison DB, Zannolli R, Faith MS, Heo M, Pietrobelli A, Van-Itallie TB, Pi-Sunyer FX, Heymsfield SB. Weight loss increases and fat loss decreases all-cause mortality rate: results from two independent cohort studies. Int J Obes 1999; 23: 603–611.

19. Barlow CE, Kohl HW 3rd, Gibbons LW, Blair SN. Physical fitness, mortality, and obesity. Int J Obes Relat Metab Disord 1995; 19: S41–S44.

20. Lee CD, Blair SN, Jackson AS. Cardiorespiratory fitness, body composition, and all-cause and cardiovascular disease mortality in men. Am J Clin Nutr 1999; 69: 373–380.

21. Wei M, Kampert JB, Barlow CE, Nichaman MZ, Gibbons LW, Paffenbarger Jr RS, Blair SN. Relationship between low cardiorespiratory fitness and mortality in normal-weight, overweight, and obese men. JAMA 1999; 282: 1547–1553.

22. Stampfer MJ, Hu FB, Manson JE, Rimm EB, Willett WC. Primary prevention of coronary heart disease in women through diet and lifestyle. N Engl J Med 2000; 343: 16–22.

23. Shike M. Body weight and colon cancer. Am J Clin Nutr 1996; 63: 442S–444S.

24. Lichtenstein P, Holm NV, Verkasalo PK, Iliadou A, Kaprio J, Koskenvou M, Pukkala E, Skytthe A, Hemminki K. Environmental and heritable factors in the causation of cancer. N Engl J Med 2000; 343: 78–85.

25. Stevens J. Impact of age on associations between weight and mortality. Nutr Rev 2000; 58: 129–137.

26. Sjöström LV. Mortality of severely obese subjects. Am J Clin Nutr 1992; 55: 516S–523S.
27. Solomon CG, Manson JE. Obesity and mortality: a review of the epidemiologic data. Am J Clin Nutr 1997; 66: 1044S–1050S.
28. Iribarren C, Sharp DS, Burchfiel CM, Petrovitch H. Association of weight loss and weight fluctuation with mortality among Japanese American men. N Engl J Med 1995; 333: 686–692.
29. Williamson DF. Intentional weight loss: patterns in the general population and its association with morbidity and mortality. Int J Obes Relat Metab Disord 1997; 21: S14–S19.
30. Williamson DF. Weight loss and mortality in persons with type 2 diabetes mellitus: a review of the epidemiologic evidence. Exp Clin Endocrinol 1998; 106: 14–21.
31. Yanovski SZ, Bain RP, Williamson DF. Report of the NIH–CDC workshop on the feasibility of conducting a randomized clinical trial to evaluate the long-term health impact of intentional weight loss in obese persons. Am J Clin Nutr 1999; 69: 366–372.
32. Williamson D, Parnuk E, Thus M, Flanders D, Byers T, Heath C. Prospective study of intentional weight loss and mortality in never-smoking overweight US white women aged 40–64. Am J Epidemiol 1995; 141: 1128–1141.
33. Kelley DE. Managing obesity as first-line therapy for diabetes mellitus. Nutr Clin Care 1998; 1: 38–43.
34. Pi-Sunyer FX. Co-morbidities for overweight and obesity: current evidence and research issues. Med Sci Sports Exerc 1999; 31: S602–S608.
35. Brown CD, Higgins M, Donato KA, Rohde FC, Garrison R, Obarzanek E, Ernst ND, Horan M. Body mass index and the prevalence of hypertension and dyslipidemia. Obes Res 2000; 8: 605–619.
36. Hubert HB, Feinbeib M, McNamara PM, Castelli W. Obesity as an independent risk factor for cardiovascular disease: a 26-year follow-up of participants in the Framingham Heart Study. Circulation 1983; 5: 968–977.
37. Garrison RJ, Castelli WP. Weight and thirty-year mortality of men in the Framingham Study. Ann Intern Med 1985; 103: 1006–1009.
38. Rimm EB, Stampler MJ, Giovannucci B, Ascherio V, Spiegelman D, Colditz GA, Willett WC. Body size and fat distribution as predictors of coronary heart disease among middle-aged and older US men. Am J Epidemiol 1995; 141: 1117–1127.
39. Després J-P. The insulin resistance–dyslipidemic syndrome

of visceral obesity: effect on patients' risk. Obes Res 1998; 6: 8S–17S.

40. Rexrode KM, Hennekens CH, Willett WC, Colditz GA, Stampfer MJ, Rich-Edwards JW, Speizer FE, Manson JE. A prospective study of body mass index, weight change and risk of a stroke in women. JAMA 1997; 277: 1539–1545.

41. Larsson B, Svardsudd K, Welin L, Wilhemsen L, Bjorntorp P, Tibblin G. Abdominal adipose distribution, obesity and risk of cardiovascular disease death: 13-year follow-up of participants in the study born in 1913. Br Med J 1984; 288: 1401–1404.

42. Shaper AG, Wannamethee SG, Walker M. Body weight: implications for the prevention of coronary heart disease, stroke, and diabetes mellitus in a cohort study of middle aged men. Br Med J 1997; 314: 1311–1317.

43. Krauss RM, Winston M. Obesity: impact on cardiovascular disease. Circulation 1998; 98: 1472–1476.

44. Heyka RJ. Obesity and hypertension. Nutr Clin Care 1998; 1: 30–37.

45. Dyer AR, Elliot P, on behalf of the INTERSALT Co-operative Research Group (1989). The INTERSALT study: relations of body mass index to blood pressure. J Hum Hypertens 1989; 3: 299–308.

46. Stepniakowski K, Egan BM. Additive effects of obesity and hypertension to limit venous volume. Am J Physiol 1995; 268: R562–R568.

47. Schotte DE, Stunkard AJ. The effects of weight reduction on blood pressure in 301 obese patients. Arch Intern Med 1990; 150: 1701–1704.

48. Stevens VJ, Corrigan SA, Obarzanek E, Bernauer E, Cook NR, Hebert P, Mattfeldt-Beman M, Oberman A, Sugars C, Dalcin AT, et al. Weight loss intervention in phase I of the Trials of Hypertension Prevention. The TOHP Collaborative Research Group. Arch Intern Med 1993; 153: 849–858.

49. National Institutes of Health, National Heart, Lung and Blood Institute, National High Blood Pressure Education Program. Sixth report of the Joint National Committee of prevention, detection, evaluation, and treatment of high blood pressure. NIH Publication No. 98–4080, November 1997.

50. Trials of Hypertension Prevention Collaborative Research Group. The effects of nonpharmacologic interventions on blood pressure of persons with high normal levels: results of the trials of hypertension prevention, phase I. JAMA 1992; 267: 1213–1220.

51. Trials of Hypertension Prevention Collaborative Research Group. Effects of weight loss and sodium reduction intervention on blood pressure and hypertension incidence in over-

weight people with high normal blood pressure: the trials of hypertension prevention, phase II. Arch Intern Med 1997; 157: 657–667.

52. Sjöström CD, Lissner L, Sjöström L. Relationships between changes in body composition and changes in cardiovascular risk factors: the Swedish Obese Subjects (SOS) intervention study. Obes Res 1997; 5: 519–530.

53. Yong LC, Kuller LH, Rutan G, Bunker C. Longitudinal study of blood pressure: changes and determinants from adolescence to middle age. Dormont High School follow-up study 1957–1963 to 1989–1990. Am J Epidemiol 1993; 138: 973–983.

54. Huang Z, Willett WC, Manson JE, Rosner B, Stampfer MJ, Speizer FE, Colditz GA. Body weight, weight change, and risk for hypertension in women. Ann Intern Med 1998; 128: 81–88.

55. National High Blood Pressure Education Program Working Group. National High Blood Pressure Education Program Working Group report on primary prevention of hypertension. Arch Intern Med 1993; 153: 186–208.

56. National Heart Lung and Blood Institute. Press statement. Washington, DC: November 15, 1995.

57. Defronzo RA, Ferrannini E. Insulin resistance: a multifaceted syndrome responsible for NIDDM, obesity, hypertension, dyslipidemia and atherosclerotic cardiovascular disease. Diabetes Care 1991; 14: 173–194.

58. Ikeda T, Gomi T, Hirawa N, Sakurai J, Yoshikawa N. Improvement of insulin sensitivity contributes to blood pressure reduction after weight loss in hypertensive subjects with obesity. Hypertension 1996; 27: 1180–1186.

59. Rocchini AP. Obesity and blood pressure regulation. In: Bray GA, Bouchard C, James WPT, eds. Handbook of Obesity. New York: Marcel Dekker, 1998: 677–695.

60. Kolanowski J. Obesity and hypertension: from pathophysiology to treatment. Int J Obes 1999; 23: 42–46.

61. Benotti PN, Bistrain B, Benotti JR, Blackburn G, Forse RA. Heart disease and hypertension in severe obesity: the benefits of weight reduction. Am J Clin Nutr 1992; 55: 586S–590S.

62. Mertens IL, Van Gaal LF. Overweight, obesity, and blood pressure: the effects of modest weight reduction. Obes Res 2000; 8: 270–278.

63. Denke MA, Sempos CT, Grundy SM. Excess body weight: an underrecognized contributor to high blood cholesterol levels in white American men. Arch Intern Med 1993; 153: 1093–1103.

64. Denke MA, Sempos CT, Grundy SM. Excess body weight: an

underrecognized contributor to dyslipidemia levels in white American women. Arch Intern Med 1994; 154: 401–410.

65. Després J-P. Abdominal obesity as an important component of insulin-resistance syndrome. Nutrition 1993; 4: 452–459.

66. Assmann G, Schulte H. Role of triglycerides in coronary artery disease: lessons from the Prospective Cardiovascular Munster Study. Am J Cardiol 1992; 70: 10H–13H.

67. Dattilo A, Kris-Etherton P. Effects of weight reduction on blood lipids and lipoproteins: a meta-analysis. Am J Clin Nutr 1992; 56: 320–328.

68. Ditschuneit HH, Flechtner-Mors M, Johnson TD, Adler G. Metabolic and weight-loss effects of a long-term dietary intervention in obese patients. Am J Clin Nutr 1999; 69: 198–202.

69. Denke MA. Cholesterol-lowering diets: a review of the evidence. Arch Intern Med 1995; 155: 17–26.

70. Yu-Poth S, Zhao G, Etherton T, Naglak M, Jonnalagadda S, Kris-Etherton PM. Effects of the National Cholesterol Education Program's Step I and Step II dietary intervention programs on cardiovascular disease risk factors: a meta-analysis. Am J Clin Nutr 1999; 69: 632–646.

71. Dengel JL, Katsel LI, Goldberg AP. Effect of an American Heart Association diet, with and without weight loss, on lipids in obese middle-aged and older men. Am J Clin Nutr 1995; 62: 715–721.

72. Colditz GA, Willett WC, Rotnitzky A, Manson JE. Weight gain as a risk factor for clinical diabetes mellitus in women. Ann Intern Med 1995; 122: 481–486.

73. Seidell J, Cigolini M, Charzewska J, Ellsigner B, DiBiases G. Fat distribution in European women: a comparison of anthropometric measurements in relation to cardiovascular risk factors. Int J Epidemiol 1990; 10: 303–308.

74. Chan JM, Rimm EB, Colditz GA, Stampfer MJ, Willett WC. Obesity, fat distribution, and weight gain as risk factors for clinical diabetes in men. Diabetes Care 1994; 17: 961–969.

75. Ohlson LO, Larsson B, Svardsudd K, Welin L, Eriksson H, Wilhelmsen L, Bjorntorp P, Tibblin G. The influence of body fat distribution on the incidence of diabetes mellitus: 13.5 years of follow-up of the participants in the study of men born in 1913. Diabetes 1985; 34: 1055–1058.

76. Meigs JB, Mittleman MA, Nathtan DM, Tofler GH, Singer DE, Murphy-Sheehy PM, Lipinska I, D'Agostino RB, Wilson PWF. Hyperinsulinemia, hyperglycemia, and impaired hemostasis: the Framingham Offspring Study. JAMA 2000; 238: 221–228.

77. Wall JR, Pyke DA, Oakley WG. Effect of carbohydrate restric-

tion in obese diabetics: relationship of control to weight loss. Br Med J 1973; 10: 577–578.

78. Liu GC, Coulston AM, Lardinois CK, Hollenbeck CB, Moore JG, Reaven GM. Moderate weight loss and sylfonylurea treatment of non-insulin-dependent diabetes mellitus. Arch Intern Med 1985; 145: 665–669.

79. Reaven GM, and staff of the Palo Alto GRECC Aging Study Unit. Beneficial effect of moderate weight loss in older patients with non-insulin-dependent diabetes mellitus poorly controlled with insulin. J Am Geriatr Soc 1985; 33: 93–95.

80. Wing RR, Koeske R, Epstein LH, Nowalk MP, Gooding W, Becker D. Long-term effects of modest weight loss in type 2 diabetic patients. Arch Intern Med 1987; 147: 1749–1753.

81. Pories WJ, MacDonald KG Jr, Morgan EJ, Sinha MK, Dohm GL, Swanson MS, Barakaat HA, Khazanie PG, Leggett-Frazier N, Long SD. Surgical treatment of obesity and its effect on diabetes: 10-year follow-up. Am J Clin Nutr 1992; 55: 582S–585S.

82. Goldstein DJ. Beneficial health effects of modest weight loss. Int J Obes 1992; 56: 320–328.

83. Moore LL, Visioni AJ, Wilson PWF, D'Agostino RB, Finkle D, Ellison RC. Can sustained weight loss in overweight individuals reduce the risk of diabetes mellitus? Epidemiology 2000; 11: 269–273.

84. Wing RR. Use of very-low-calorie diets in the treatment of obese persons with non-insulin-dependent diabetes mellitus. J Am Diet Assoc 1995; 95: 569–572.

85. Van Gaal LF, Wauters MA, De Leeus IH. The beneficial effect of modest weight loss on cardiovascular risk factors. Int J Obes 1997; 21: 5S–9S.

86. Ditschuneit HH, Fletchtner-Mors M, Asler G. Fibrinogen in obesity before and after weight reduction. Obes Res 1995; 3: 43–49.

87. Folsom AR, Qamhieh HT, Wing RR, Jeffery RW, Stinson VL, Kuller LH, Wu KK. Impact of weight loss on plasminogen activator inhibitor (PAI-1), factor VII, and other hemostatic factors in moderately overweight adults. Arterioscler Thromb 1993; 13: 162–169.

88. Marckmann P, Toubro S, Astrup A. Sustained improvement in blood lipids, coagulation, and fibrinolysis after major weight loss in obese subjects. Eur J Clin Nutr 1998; 52: 329–333.

89. Yusuf HR, Giles WH, Croft JB, Anda RF, Casper ML. Impact of multiple risk factor profiles on determining cardiovascular disease risk. Prev Med 1998; 27: 1–9.

90. World Health Organization. MONICA Project: risk factors. Int J Epidemiol 1989; 18: S46–S55.

91. Wilson PWF, Kannel WB, Silbershatz H, D'Agostino RB.

Clustering of metabolic factors and coronary heart disease. Arch Intern Med 1999; 159: 1104–1109.

92. Prineas R, Flosom A, Kaye S. Central adiposity and increased risk of coronary artery mortality in older women. Ann Epidemiol 1993; 3: 35–41.

93. Freedman D, Williams D, Croft J, Ballew C, Byers T. Relation of body fat distribution to ischemic heart disease: the National Health and Nutrition Examination Survey I (NHANES I) epidemiologic follow-up study. Am J Epidemiol 1995; 142: 53–63.

94. Terry R, Page W, Haskell W. Waist/hip ratio, body mass indexes and premature cardiovascular mortality in US Army during a 23-year follow up study. Int J Obes 1992; 16: 417–423.

95. Despres J-P, Lamarche B, Mauriege P, Cantin B, Dagenais GR, Moorjani S, Lupien P-J. Hyperinsulinemia as an independent risk factor for ischemic heart disease. N Engl J Med 1996; 334: 952–957.

96. Despres J-P. Dyslipidemia and obesity. Baillieres Best Pract Clin Endocrinol Metab 1994; 8: 629–660.

97. Lemieux S, Despres J-P, Moorjani S, Nadeau A, Theriault G, Prud'homme D, Tremblay A, Bouchard C, Lupien PJ. Are gender differences in cardiovascular disease risk factors explained by the level of visceral adipose tissue? Diabetologia 1994; 37: 757–764.

98. Rissnanen P, Hamalainen P, Vanninen E, Tenhunen-Eskelinen M, Uusitupa M. Relationship of metabolic variables to abdominal adiposity measured by different anthropometric measurements and dual-energy X-ray absorptiometry in obese middle-aged women. Int J Obes Relat Metab Disord 1997; 21: 367–371.

99. Pietrobelli A, Lee RC, Capristo E, Deckelbaum RJ, Heymsfield SB. An independent, inverse association of high-density-lipoprotein-cholesterol concentration with nonadipose body mass. Am J Clin Nutr 1999; 69: 614–620.

100. Pouliot MC, Despres J-P, Nadeau A, Moorjani S, Prud'homme D, Lupien P-J, Tremblay A, Bouchard C. Visceral obesity in men: associations with glucose tolerance, plasma insulin, and lipoprotein levels. Diabetes 1992; 41: 826–834.

101. Kanaley JA, Anderson-Reid ML, Oenning L, Kottke BA, Jenson MD. Different health benefits of weight loss in upper-body and lower-body obese women. Am J Clin Nutr 1993; 57: 20–26.

102. Ross R, Janssen I. Is abdominal fat preferentially reduced in response to exercise-induced weight loss? Med Sci Sports Exerc 1999; 31: S568–S572.

103. Smith SR, Zachwieja JJ. Visceral adipose tissue: a critical review of intervention strategies. Int J Obes 1999; 23: 329–335.

104. Pi-Sunyer FX. Short-term medical benefits and adverse effects of weight loss. Ann Intern Med 1993; 119: 772–776.

105. Tremblay A, Doucet E, Imbeault P, Mauriege P, Despres J-P, Richard D. Metabolic fitness in active reduced-obese individuals. Obes Res 1999; 7: 556–563.

106. Gleysteen JJ, Barboriak JJ, Sasse EA. Sustained coronary-risk-factor reduction after gastric bypass for morbid obesity. Am J Clin Nutr 1990; 51: 774–778.

107. Wadden TA, Anderson DA, Foster GD. Two-year changes in lipids and lipoproteins associated with the maintenance of a 5–10% reduction in initial weight: some findings and some questions. Obes Res 1999; 7: 170–178.

108. Mancini M, Giuseppe DB, Contalso F, Fischetti A, Grasso L, Mattioli P. Medical complications of severe obesity: importance of treatment by very-low-calorie diets: intermediate and long-term effects. Int J Obes 1981; 5: 34–352.

109. Wing RR, Marcus MD, Salata R, Epstein LH, Miaskiewicz S, Blair EH. Effects of a very low-calorie diet on a long-term glycemic control in obese type II diabetic subjects. Arch Intern Med 1991; 151: 1334–1440.

110. Hensrud DD, Weinsier RL, Darnell BE, Hunter GR. Relationships of co-morbidities of obesity to weight loss and 4-year weight maintenance/rebound. Obes Res 1995; 3: 217S–222S.

111. Garfinkel L. Overweight and cancer. Ann Intern Med 1985; 103: 1034–1036.

112. Ballard-Barbash R, Swanson CA. Body weight: estimation of risk for breast and endometrial cancers. Am J Clin Nutr 1996; 63: 437S–441S.

113. Huang Z, Hankinson SE, Colditz GA, Stampfer MJ, Hunter DJ, Manson JE, Hennekens CH, Rosner B, Speizer FE, Willett WC. Dual effects of weight and weight gain on breast cancer risk. JAMA 1997; 278: 1407–1411.

114. Anderson JJ, Felson DT. Factors associated with osteoarthritis of the knee in the first National Health and Nutrition Examination Survey (NHANES I): evidence for an association with overweight, race, and physical demands of work. Am J Epidemiol 1988; 128: 179–189.

115. Davis MA, Ettinger WH, Neuhaus JM, Cho SA, Hauck WW. The association of knee injury and obesity with unilateral and bilateral osteoarthritis of the knee. Am J Epidemiol 1989; 130: 278–288.

116. Felson DT. Weight and osteoarthritis. Am J Clin Nutr 1996; 63: 430S–432S.

117. Hochberg MC, Lethbridge-Cejku M. Epidemiologic considerations in the primary prevention of osteoarthritis. In: Hamerman D, ed. Osteoarthritis: public health implications for an aging population. Baltimore: Johns Hopkins University Press, 1997: 169–186.

118. Toda Y, Toda T, Takemura S, Wada T, Morimoto T, Ogawa R. Change in body fat, but not body weight or metabolic correlates of obesity, is related to symptomatic relief or obese patients with knee osteoarthritis after a weight control program. J Rheumatol 1998; 25: 2181–2186.

119. Hart DJ, Spector TD. The relationship of obesity, fat distribution and osteoarthritis in women in the general population: the Chingford Study. J Rheumatol 1993; 20: 331–335.

120. Felson DT, Zhang Y, Anthony JM, Naimark A, Anderson JJ. Weight loss reduces the risk for symptomatic knee osteoarthritis in women: the Framingham study. Ann Intern Med 1992; 16: 116–117.

121. Guilleminault C, Quera-Salva MA, Partinen M, Jamieson A. Women and the obstructive sleep apnea syndrome. Chest 1988; 93: 104–109.

122. Young T, Palta M, Dempsey J, Skatrud J, Weber S, Badr S. The occurrence of sleep-disordered breathing among middle-aged adults. N Engl J Med 1993; 328: 1230–1235.

123. Vgontzas AN, Tan TL, Bixler EO, Martin LF, Shubert D, Kales A. Sleep apnea and sleep disruption in obese patients. Arch Intern Med 1994; 154: 1705–1711.

124. Strohl KP, Strobel RJ, Parisi RA. Obesity and pulmonary function. In: Bray GA, Bouchard C, James WPT, eds. Handbook of obesity. New York, NY: Marcel Dekker, 1998: 725–739.

125. Charuzi I, Lavie P, Peiser J, Peled R. Bariatric surgery in morbidly obese sleep-apnea patients: short- and long-term follow-up. Am J Clin Nutr 1992; 55: 594S–596S.

126. Sugerman HJ, Fairman RP, Sood RK, Engle K, Wolfe L, Kellum JM. Long-term effects of gastric surgery for treating respiratory insufficiency of obesity. Am J Clin Nutr 1992; 55: 597S–601S.

127. Kodama H, Kono S, Todoroki I, Honjo S, Sakurai Y, Wakabayashi K, Nishiwaki M, Hamada H, Nishikawa H, Koga H, Ogawa S, Nakagawa K. Gallstone disease risk in relation to body mass index and waist-to-hip ratio in Japanese men. Int J Obes Relat Metab Disord 1999; 23: 211–216.

128. Kato I, Nomura A, Stemmermann GN, Chyou PH. Prospective study of clinical gallbladder disease and its association with obesity, physical activity, and other factors. Dig Dis Sci 1992; 37: 784–790.

129. Stampfer MJ, Maclure KM, Colditz GA, Manson JE, Willett WC. Risk of symptomatic gallstones in women with severe obesity. Am J Clin Nutr 1992; 55: 652–658.

130. Andersen T. Liver and gallbladder disease before and after very-low-calorie diets. Am J Clin Nutr 1992; 56: 235S–239S.

131. Sheth SG, Gordon FD, Chopra S. Non-alcoholic steathohepatitis. Ann Intern Med 1997; 126: 137–145.

132. Eriksson S, Eriksson KF, Bondesson L. Non-alcoholic steatohepatitis in obesity: a reversible condition. Acta Medica Scand 1986; 220: 83–88.

133. National Cholesterol Education Program. Report of the expert panel on detection, evaluation, and treatment of high blood cholesterol in adults. Washington, DC: US Department of Health and Human Services, 1993.

134. National Institutes of Health (NIH). Consensus development conference on diet and exercise in non-insulin dependent diabetes mellitus. Diabetes Care 1987; 10: 639–644.

135. Sager D. Diet, behavior modification, and exercise: a review of obesity treatments from a long-term perspective. South Med J 1991; 84: 1470–1474.

136. Rippe JM. The obesity epidemic: a mandate for a multidisciplinary approach. JAMA 1998; 98: S1–S64.

137. Pasman WJ, Saris WHM, Westerterp-Plantenga MS. Predictors of weight maintenance. Obes Res 1999; 7: 43–50.

138. Klem M, Wing R, McGuire M, Seagle H, Hill J. A descriptive study of individuals successful at long-term maintenance of substantial weight loss. Am J Clin Nutr 1997; 66: 239–246.

139. McGuire MT, Wing RR, Klem ML, Hill JO. Behavioral strategies of individuals who have maintained long-term weight losses. Obes Res 1999; 7: 334–341.

140. Klem ML, Wing RR, Lang W, McGuire MT, Hill JO. Does weight loss maintenance become easier over time? Obes Res 2000; 8: 438–444.

Chapter 8

Childhood Obesity

Scott Owens and Bernard Gutin

The prevalence of childhood obesity has increased dramatically in the United States and other industrialized nations during the past two to three decades. While the social and psychological burdens often encountered by obese children might seem like challenge enough, there is the additional issue of the short- and long-term medical consequences of their obesity. Because it is likely that pediatricians and other health care professionals will have increasingly frequent treatment opportunities with obese children, it is important to stay abreast of the latest research in the field.

In this chapter we present an overview of the current state of knowledge regarding childhood obesity. Issues related to the definition and prevalence of childhood obesity are discussed first. In the next section, the implications of childhood obesity are presented, emphasizing the notion that many adult diseases have their beginnings in childhood. The etiology of childhood obesity is discussed next, with special emphasis on the importance of the physical activity component of energy expenditure. The final section presents the most recent findings regarding the treatment of childhood obesity, including data that suggest that there is cause for optimism regarding long-term outcomes.

DEFINITION AND PREVALENCE OF CHILDHOOD OBESITY

Defining childhood obesity is difficult, and no generally accepted definition has yet emerged (1,2). Ideally, the definition should reflect adiposity, or the amount of body fat, and be related to morbidity and mortality outcomes. An ideal measure of body fat would be:

1. accurate in its measure of body fat;
2. precise, with a small measurement error;
3. accessible, in terms of simplicity, cost, and ease of use;
4. acceptable to the subject; and
5. have published reference values (3).

Unfortunately, no current measure satisfies all these criteria. Highly accurate methods such as isotope dilution or magnetic resonance imaging (MRI) are useful research tools, but are expensive and generally impractical in clinical settings. Underwater densitometry, also widely used in adult research, requires considerable time and subject cooperation, making it less desirable for use with children. These drawbacks have resulted in the continued reliance on anthropometric measurements in the clinical setting. Although not the ideal measures of adiposity for every individual, anthropometric measures tend to satisfy the criteria of simplicity, cost, ease of use, and availability of reference values. Some frequently encountered anthropometric definitions of childhood obesity include body weight greater than 120% predicted from height (4), body mass index (BMI) greater than the 85th percentile (1), triceps skinfold thickness greater than the 85th percentile (5), and a body fat level higher than 25% for boys and 30% for girls as estimated from the sum of subscapular and triceps skinfolds (6). Several authors have recommended BMI as the measurement of choice for most clinical settings because of its high reliability and ease of measurement (3,7).

Prevalence data from the third National Health and Nutrition Examination Survey (NHANES III, 1988–1991), which used the 85th percentile of BMI from previous national samples as the reference point, estimated the prevalence of child (ages 6–11) and adolescent (ages 12–17) obesity for all race and ethnic groups combined to be 22% (1). Data from this nationally representative cross-sectional survey clearly indicate a dramatic increase in the prevalence of excess body mass in relation to height in children and adolescents in the United States since the mid-1960s. Obesity prevalence increased among all sex and age groups. Similarly, increased ponderosity (weight/height^3) has been reported for cohorts of children examined between 1973 and 1992 in the Bogalusa Heart Study (8). Trends for increased obesity in children also have been observed in other industrialized countries, including France (9), and England and Scotland (10). It is likely, therefore, that pediatricians will encounter the obese child on a routine basis.

IMPLICATIONS OF CHILDHOOD OBESITY

Although obesity-related health problems such as coronary artery disease (CAD), hypertension, and non-insulin-dependent diabetes mellitus (NIDDM) tend to present their clinical manifestations in adulthood, evidence indicates these disorders have their beginnings in childhood (11), with obese children tending to have a poorer risk profile for these diseases than their counterparts of normal weight. Childhood obesity is associated with elevated levels of triglycerides (8,12) and low-density lipoprotein (LDL) cholesterol (13), and reduced levels of high-density lipoprotein (HDL) cholesterol (8,14). Obese children tend to display higher levels of blood pressure (15,16) and insulin (12,13) than non-obese children. In adults, the clustering of risk factors such as dyslipidemia, hypertension, and hyperinsulinemia is often referred to as "Syndrome X" or the insulin-resistance syndrome; it places an individual at an unusually high risk for CAD and NIDDM (17). For children, data from the Bogalusa Heart Study indicate the clustering of the Syndrome X risk factors begins around age 5, that the clustering tracks from childhood into young adulthood, and tracks more strongly in obese children (11).

Several other worrisome associations with childhood obesity have been reported recently. In a group of lean and obese children, higher percentages of body fat were associated with increased left ventricular mass and relative wall thickness (the ratio of left ventricular wall thickness to cavity size) and with decreased left ventricular mid-wall fractional shortening (18). In adults, greater left ventricular mass and relative wall thickness are predictive of future cardiovascular morbidity (19). Decreased mid-wall fractional shortening is an index of left ventricular systolic function that identifies individuals at elevated risk for future cardiovascular mortality who are otherwise undetected by conventional endocardial shortening indices (20). Also, in a group of 7- to 13-year-old children, increased body fat was associated with greater endothelial dysfunction as represented by a lower amount of femoral artery dilatation in response to the increased blood flow that occurred following the release of a tourniquet (21). Endothelial dysfunction is a relatively early event in atherogenesis (22). More specifically, low levels of endothelium-dependent arterial dilatation are associated with various manifestations of cardiovascular disease in adults and children (23). These results support the idea that fatness plays a part in the early stages of the atherogenic process.

In addition to overall adiposity, fat patterning in childhood obesity may have implications. In adults, fat stored in the abdominal region, especially in the visceral compartment, is more clearly associated with Syndrome X and the development of CAD and NIDDM than is fat stored in other parts of the body (24–26). Some (27,28), but not all (12), studies of children have detected an association between fat patterning and risk factors. An important limitation of child studies that used anthropometry or dual X-ray absorptiometry (DXA) is that they could not distinguish subcutaneous abdominal adipose tissue from the more deleterious visceral adipose tissue. In adults, various measures of central fat deposition, including the waist:hip ratio or waist circumference alone, may be related to risk factors. However, in children, very little of the abdominal fat is in the visceral adipose tissue compartment relative to the amount in subcutaneous abdominal adipose tissue (29,30). Therefore, at an early stage in the development of Syndrome X (i.e. in childhood), it may be necessary to measure visceral adipose tissue directly in order to uncover its relation to other risk factors. In this regard, a study that used MRI in obese children found that visceral adipose tissue, but not subcutaneous abdominal adipose tissue, was significantly related to LDL cholesterol and triglycerides (30). Furthermore, a study involving obese and non-obese adolescent girls found that visceral adipose tissue was significantly correlated with triglycerides, HDL cholesterol, and insulin in the obese girls only (31). On the other hand, a study of non-obese 7- to 10-year-old girls found no significant relationship between visceral adipose tissue and triglycerides, HDL cholesterol, or insulin (32). Therefore, the visceral adipose tissue–risk factor relationship appears to be more pronounced in obese than in lean children. From a clinical perspective, it is not yet clear the extent to which visceral adiposity can be predicted from the anthropometric measurements commonly used in clinical settings.

Not to be overlooked is evidence that childhood obesity is often associated with significant social and psychological problems. In a study of 139 obese and 150 non-obese children aged 9–12, the obese children reported more negative physical self-perceptions than their non-obese peers and scored lower on measures of general self-worth (33). Studies show that obese children report more depression and receive more negative peer reactions than non-obese children (34,35). When shown drawings of six children, four with physical disabilities, one with no physical disability, and an obese child, both children and adults rated the obese child as the least likable (36,37). It is likely that the immediacy of the social and psychological implications of obesity is of greater concern to children than the long-term health implications.

ETIOLOGY OF CHILDHOOD OBESITY

Childhood obesity is the result of a complex interaction of genetic and environmental factors. In a recent review of the role of genes in the variation of human body mass, two of the conclusions were:

1. there are good reasons to believe that the genes involved in body mass variation over time in a given individual as well as those responsible for population heterogeneity in body mass eventually will be identified; and

2. there are equally good reasons to believe that environmental conditions and lifestyle characteristics make an even stronger contribution than the genes to intra-individual and inter-individual variation in body mass (38).

Regardless of whether the underlying impetus is genetic or environmental, it is understood that obesity results from an imbalance between energy intake and energy expenditure.

Energy Intake

It is evident that accurate and reliable quantitative information about energy and macronutrient intake would be valuable, but such data are difficult to obtain, especially in children. Cross-sectional studies using diet recall methods generally have not found a relationship between body fatness and energy intake (39). These results are counterintuitive, in light of the fact that obese adults and children have relatively high fat-free mass along with their elevated fat mass, and consequently have elevated resting energy expenditure (40), the largest component of 24-h energy expenditure. Assuming that the energy costs of thermoregulation and growth are small (41), 24-h energy expenditure must equal energy intake. Using the doubly labeled water procedure (i.e. isotope dilution) to validate self-reported measures of energy intake, it has been found that obese adults (42) and adolescents (43) tend to underreport energy intake to a greater degree than lean people. More objective and expensive means of collecting diet data, such as direct observation, might influence the youth's diet behavior and are very intrusive; thus this methodology is not feasible for most studies. Consequently, methodological considerations make it difficult to draw any clear conclusions about the role of total free living energy intake in the etiology of obesity.

Perhaps these methodological difficulties partly explain why it is difficult to find evidence that the increased prevalence of childhood obesity over the past few decades is the result of increased caloric intake. In fact, the reported mean daily energy intakes of 6- to 11-year-olds showed a slight decline (3%) from NHANES II (1976–80) to NHANES III (1988–91) (44). In another study, the daily caloric intakes of 1670 (1977–1978) and 1463 (1986–88) of children aged 2–10 remained constant over the 10-year period, with mean intakes of 1632 kcal in 1978 and 1613 kcal in 1988 (45).

With respect to fat intake, most (46–48), but not all, studies (49) support the idea that diets high in fat are associated with body fatness or gain in weight. Lissner et al (50) found that a high-fat diet led to greater 6-year weight gain in women who were sedentary, but not in those who were physically active. Thus, it may be the synergistic effect of a high-fat diet and sedentary behavior that is a key determinant of obesity. Prospective studies testing this hypothesis have not yet been reported in children.

Energy Expenditure

Total energy expenditure is comprised of resting metabolic rate, the thermic effect of food, and physical activity; resting metabolic rate constitutes 60–70% of the total, the thermic effect of food approximately 10%, and physical activity the remainder.

Resting Metabolic Rate

A cross-sectional study found that children of obese parents had relatively low resting metabolic rates (51), suggesting that they were at increased risk for development of obesity. However, when these children were followed up 12 years later (52), the children of the obese parents were not found to be more obese than the children of non-obese parents. Moreover, two larger scale doubly labeled water studies

(41,53) failed to find any evidence that children of obese parents had defects in any aspect of energy expenditure.

Cross-sectional studies comparing obese and non-obese children, in which the influence of body composition was taken into account statistically, have found the groups to have similar resting and 24-h metabolic rates (43,54,55). However, the cross-sectional nature of these investigations precludes firm conclusions of causality; prospective studies in children of different ages are needed to elucidate the nature of these relationships. In this regard, a recent doubly labeled water study of children (56) failed to show that resting energy expenditure predicted body fatness 2–4 years later. Therefore, there is little reason to believe that variation in resting metabolic rate explains the development of childhood obesity.

Thermic Effect of Food In order to capture most of the thermic effect of food it is necessary to measure postprandial metabolism while the child remains relatively motionless for several hours, a daunting task for both the subjects and investigators. Moreover, the thermic effect of food is the component of energy expenditure which is least reproducible (57). Therefore, it has not been extensively studied and its role in the etiology of childhood obesity is unclear. Although some adult studies suggest that the thermic effect of food may be blunted in obese people (58), cross-sectional studies of children do not provide a consistent picture concerning differences between lean and obese populations (43,54) and no prospective studies in children have been reported.

Physical Activity Although physical activity constitutes a relatively small portion of total energy expenditure on average, it has potential importance in explaining obesity development for several reasons.

1. It is largely volitional.
2. Its great individual variability provides an opportunity for it to explain a large portion of the variance in total energy expenditure.

3. Activity can increase fat-free mass, the main determinant of resting metabolic rate (59), with long-term consequences on energy balance.

4. Exercise training can influence substrate utilization, thereby playing a part in how ingested nutrients are partitioned into fat and fat-free mass.

It is problematic to determine from non-experimental studies whether exercise and body fatness are related because of the difficulty of knowing how to express physical activity. If it is expressed as energy expenditure, then it might be concluded that obese youths are more active than lean youths, as was found in a doubly labeled water study by Bandini et al (43). However, differences in mechanical work done must be considered when interpreting data on energy expenditure during activity; i.e. a heavier child uses more energy to move the body a given distance. Thus, if a lean and an obese child display the same free-living activity energy expenditure, it represents less movement in the obese child. Consequently, it is necessary to adjust activity energy expenditure for body weight to determine if variations in movement are associated with fatness. The problem concerns the exponent to use in making this adjustment. If an exponent of one is used—i.e. energy expenditure is simply divided by weight—then an overcorrection may result, automatically creating a negative correlation with fatness (59). Unfortunately, the correction factor varies for different children, depending on how much of their activity involves carrying the body weight (e.g. walking/running) and how much involves activity in which the body weight is supported and most of the work is external (e.g. cycling). The variety of procedures used to try to correct for body weight may account for the discrepant findings of cross-sectional doubly labeled water studies (41,60,61).

Unfortunately, perhaps for some of these same reasons, prospective studies that have used doubly labeled water methodology have not provided a clear picture either. One study (62) suggested that greater activity energy expenditure led to less weight gain during the first year of life in a small group of infants, but a larger scale study (56) failed to show that activity energy expenditure predicted body fatness 2–4 years later.

Time–motion studies, even those that depend on self or parental report (which is less objective than energy expenditure measurements) may provide a more direct index of how much actual exercise the child does. Cross-sectional studies of this nature show that active children are less fat (61) even while ingesting more energy (63); however, it is impossible to tell whether the activity caused less fatness or whether lower fatness caused the greater activity. A clearer picture emerges from recent epidemiologic studies in which the exercise levels of children were estimated by the parents in relation to other children of the same age. It was found that lower exercise levels and family history of obesity were principal risk factors for later development of childhood obesity (64) or higher levels of BMI (65). Another recent study, which used the Caltrac movement sensor to measure activity, found that preschoolers who were classified as inactive were 3.8 times as likely as active children to have an increasing triceps skinfold slope during the average of 2.5 years of follow-up (66).

The childhood behavior most frequently cited as contributing to increased physical inactivity is television watching. In a recent study, Gortmaker et al (67) examined the relationship between hours of television viewed and the prevalence of overweight in 1990, and the incidence of overweight from 1986 to 1990 in a nationally representative sample of 746 youths from the ages of 10 to 15. Overweight was defined as BMI greater than the 85th percentile for age and gender. The study reported a strong dose–response relationship between the prevalence of overweight in 1990 and hours of television viewed. After controlling for potentially confounding variables such as previous overweight status, household structure, socioeconomic status, maternal overweight, and ethnicity, the odds of being overweight were 5.3 times greater for youth watching more than 5 h/day of television compared with those watching 2 h or less. The investigators also examined prospectively the association of variables measured in 1986 with television viewing in 1990. In a multivariate regression predicting television viewing, they found no evidence that causality was running in the opposite than suggested direction, i.e. that being overweight was a cause of television viewing. Analysis of television viewing data from NHANES III (4069 children aged 8–16 years) revealed that children who watched the most number of hours of television per day had the highest prevalence of obesity; this held true after controlling for age, race/ethnicity, and family income (68). In a study of younger children (aged 3–4), on the other hand, television viewing time was not related to fatness (69). A possible explanation for these divergent findings is that the effects of television viewing on weight are likely to be small in the short term, but to be cumulative across time. By age 10–15, the effect of television on increased fatness has had many years to take effect (67). Along these lines, Goran (70) has noted that the average energy imbalance responsible for fat gain in children is generally very small (approximately 30 kcal/day), or the equivalent of 15 min of television watching rather than play.

To the degree that aerobic fitness can be accepted as a proxy for physical activity, recent results of a 3-year longitudinal study of 7- to 12-year-olds (71) are pertinent. It was found that those children who increased the most in maximal oxygen consumption were those who increased the most in fat-free mass but increased the least in skinfold fatness. In a similar vein, Johnson et al (72) examined predictors of increasing adiposity across 3–5 years in a group of 95 white and African American children. Although initial fat mass was the main predictor of increasing adiposity, they also observed a significant negative relationship between aerobic fitness and the rate of increasing adiposity. With every increase of 0.1 L/min in maximal oxygen consumption, there was a decrease of 0.081 kg fat per kg of lean mass gained.

Another factor to consider is the intensity of the activity. In adults, Tremblay et al (73) found that when total energy expenditure during physical activity was held constant statistically, people who engaged in high-intensity exercise were leaner and had less central fat deposition. However, little is known about the role of different exercise intensities in the etiology of childhood fatness.

Exercise may also influence accumulation of fat by improving the use of lipids as a substrate for energy (74,75), because fat oxidation has been identified as a risk factor for weight gain in adult Pima Indians (76). People who oxidized less fat than carbohydrate over the course of the day, as indicated by higher respiratory exchange ratios, were more likely to gain weight and fat mass; i.e. the unoxidized fat was more likely to go into storage. This effect was independent of 24-h energy expenditure measured in the metabolic chamber. However, the ability of lipid oxidation to predict future changes in fatness of children has not yet been elucidated in prospective studies.

In light of the recent discovery in mice that the hormone leptin decreases energy intake and increases energy expenditure, some investigations of these relations have been undertaken in children. Caprio et al (77) found in children and young adults that leptin was closely correlated with subcutaneous abdominal adipose tissue ($r = 0.84$; $P < 0.001$) and somewhat less closely correlated with visceral adipose tissue ($r = 0.59$; $P < 0.001$); in addition, acute increases in insulin concentrations did not affect circulating insulin levels. Lahlou et al (78) found that serum leptin levels were positively correlated with fasting insulin levels, adiposity, and weight gain the previous year, but were not associated with resting energy expenditure. Moreover, leptin was not related to lower energy intake; indeed, the obese children ingested 2–3 times more energy (measured with self-reports) than the lean children. Salbe et al (79) examined cross-sectional relations among these factors in 5-year-old Pima Indian children. They found that leptin concentrations, which were closely correlated to percentage body fat ($r = 0.84$; $P < 0.001$), were also correlated with physical activity level (the ratio of total:resting energy expenditure, measured with doubly labeled water), after adjustment for body fat ($r = 0.26$; $P < 0.01$). Nagy et al (80) found black and white girls to have higher leptin levels than black and white boys; however, these differences were no longer significant after controlling for total body composition, visceral adipose tissue, and subcutaneous abdominal adipose tissue. These results indicate that in children leptin is a marker of adiposity, but does not suppress energy intake or halt fat deposition, suggesting some type of leptin resistance. Perhaps the most important lesson to derive is that predictions from mouse studies concerning what relations may exist in humans must be made with great caution.

In brief, the difficulty of measuring activity and diet, compounded by the uncertainty of what is meant by "physical activity", make few definitive conclusions warranted. Perhaps the most reasonable conclusion is similar to one reached in a study of 10-year weight changes in a national cohort of adults (81); i.e. that low physical activity leads to weight gain, while weight gain leads to further diminution of activity. This would imply that interventions that either decrease fatness or increase activity would turn the cycle in the other, more favorable, direction.

Specific Endocrine and Genetic Disorders

Although specific endocrine and genetic disorders appear to be responsible for less than 10% of childhood obesity, it has been suggested that physicians rule them out as causes because they require different modes of therapy (4). Endocrine disorders to consider include Cushing's syndrome, hypothyroidism, and pseudohypoparathyroidism. Syndromes of genetic origin associated with childhood obesity include Prader–Willi, Alström, Laurence–Moon–Biedl, Carpenter, and Cohen.

TREATMENT OF CHILDHOOD OBESITY

To begin with, some researchers have cautioned against the use of treatments for obesity in children under the age of 3 whose parents are not obese (82,83). These children are at low risk of obesity in young adulthood (83). On the other hand, interventions may be warranted in obese children as young as age 1–2 if one or both parents are obese. For children who are candidates for treatment, interventions typically include diet and/or exercise. Although dieting alone can result in significant short-term weight loss in obese children, it tends to reduce fat-free mass and resting energy expenditure (84), thereby setting the stage for regain of the lost fat when the diet stops (85). On the other hand, adult studies show that exercise has the potential to reduce the diet-induced loss of fat-free mass (86). In children, the extent to which exercise alone can influence obesity is unclear. School-based interventions, where it is difficult to control and document the exercise stimulus, show mixed results for the effects of exercise on obesity status (87–89). In more highly controlled studies, where the exercise stimulus was well-documented and body fat was measured with DXA, exercise without dietary intervention resulted in significant reductions in body fat (90,91). However, the absolute amount of fat loss attained with exercise alone was modest. Therefore, a combination of exercise and diet seems more sensible for clinical use.

In this regard, one of the more promising treatment models integrates improved nutrition, increased physical activity, and behavioral modification within the context of a parental or family-based intervention. Epstein (92) has outlined the rationale for family-based behavioral interventions for obese children, noting that just as the family environment can contribute to the development of childhood obesity, it can also function as the focal point for the solution. Parenting styles influence the development of food preferences and the ability of the child to regulate intake. Parents and other family members arrange a common environment that may be conducive to overeating or a sedentary lifestyle. They also serve as role models and reinforcers for eating and exercise behaviors.

Components of Family-Based Behavioral Interventions

The basic structure of family-based behavioral interventions for childhood obesity tend to be similar; i.e. an initial short-term treatment phase followed by a longer term maintenance or continued improvement phase. During initial treatment, children typically meet in group settings once per week for 45–90 min (93,94) for between 8 (95,96) and 16 weeks (93,94,97). Facilitators for the treatment sessions have included pediatricians, child psychologists, nutritionists, and "trained therapists" (93,98–100). Follow-up sessions usually occur once (93,99) or twice per month (96,97) for 6 months to 1 year. In some cases, parents and children attend the same treatment sessions (93), but more often attend concurrent sessions (96–98). Brownell et al (93) have suggested that in older children and adolescents, having parents and offspring meet concurrently but separately may result in better long-term outcomes. Separate sessions allow for a more open discussion of sensitive issues by both parents and children and help children assume more responsibility for their treatment. Younger children may require more supervision from their parents, and this warrants holding treatment sessions together.

The specific dietary and physical activity interventions vary from study to study, as do the particular behavior modification techniques introduced. Table 8-1 summarizes this information from several family-based behavioral interventions. The variety of behavior modification methods reflects recognition of the multicomponent nature of obesity treatment and the importance of parental/family involvement.

A number of dietary approaches have been employed: some focusing on healthy eating habits rather than energy restriction, others prescribing significant caloric reduction. As an example of the latter, Figueroa-Colon et al (98) utilized a protein-sparing modified fast diet (600–800 kcal/day) for 10 weeks with obese 7- to 11-year-olds on an outpatient basis (with close medical supervision). Subsequently, the subjects transitioned to a hypocaloric balanced diet of 1200 kcal/day for the next 42 months. Although positive results were reported (see Table 8-1), others have suggested that restrictive diets be reserved for massively obese adolescents, or for children and adolescents with morbid complications of obesity, such as hypertension, sleep apnea, or NIDDM (101). Gill (102) recommends only small reductions in energy intake as a part of treatment, suggesting that excessive energy restriction in obese children is unwise and unsafe.

Epstein et al (97) have utilized a nutritional approach labeled the "traffic light" diet. This diet divides food into five categories: fruits and vegetables; grain; milk and dairy; protein; and other. Each category is subdivided into red, yellow, and green designations. These colors have the same

Table 8-1 Behavior, Diet, and Physical Activity Modifications from Selected Family-Based Behavioral Interventions for Childhood Obesity

Study	Year	Ages (yr)	Behavior Modification	Diet	Physical Activity
Brownell et al (93)	1983	12–16	Self-monitoring, stimulus control and cue elimination, behavior chains and preplanning, attitude restructuring and cognitive control, engendering family support	Nutrition education, emphasis on low sugar, salt and fat	Increasing physical activity encouraged
Figueroa-Colon et al (98)	1993	7–17	Self-monitoring, stimulus control, cue elimination, behavior chains and preplanning, using an aerobic points system, cognitive restructuring, goal setting, parent–child contracting	Hypocaloric diets (600–800 kcals/day for 10 weeks); 1200 kcals/day for next 42 weeks	Gradually increase physical activity

Study	Year	Age	Behavioral intervention	Diet	Activity
Epstein et al (97)	1995	8–12	Self-monitoring, stimulus control, reinforcement including record keeping for diet and physical activity and reciprocal contracting by parents and children	Traffic light diet with target of 1000–1200 cal/day	Subjects reinforced for either increasing physical activity or reducing sedentary behavior
Braet et al (99)	1997	7–16	Self-instruction, self-observation, self-evaluation, self-reward, behavior rehearsal, contracting, family reinforcement	Nutrition education with emphasis on eating healthy rather than eating less; no counting calories	Moderate intensity exercise for 30 min/day plus lifestyle changes to increase activity
Johnson et al (94)	1997	8–16	Cognitive/behavioral approach including contracting, self-monitoring and family support	Modified traffic light diet	Gradual increase in daily exercise up to 45 min/session, 5–7 days/week, at 60–80% of max HR

meaning as they do on a traffic light: stop (red), approach with caution (yellow), and go (green). Red foods are those high in fat or simple carbohydrates, high in calories, and low in nutrient density. Yellow foods are the staples of the diet and supply basic nutrition. Green foods are those that are lower than 20 kcal per average serving, and are represented only in the fruit and vegetable and other (condiments) groups. Children (and overweight parents) are instructed to consume between 1000 and 1200 kcal/day, to limit "red" foods to seven or fewer per week, and to maintain nutrient balance by eating the recommended servings using the eating right pyramid or the basic four food groups. However, some consider the traffic light diet too structured and limited, and instead recommend a "healthy lifestyle" approach to eating habits where counting calories is not allowed (100).

The nature of the physical activity component covers a considerable range of possibilities. Included here are general recommendations such as exercising for 30 min/day in combination with lifestyle changes (taking the stairs, walking instead of going by car, etc.) (99) to the quite specific instruction to increase aerobic exercise according to a graded 7-week schedule, up to 45 min 5–7 days/week at 60–80% of maximum heart rate (94). A novel approach to physical activity was developed by Epstein et al (97) in which children were reinforced for decreasing sedentary behavior rather than for increasing physical activity *per se*. Children who were reinforced for decreasing sedentary behavior increased their liking for high-intensity activity and reported lower caloric intake more than did children in the group that was reinforced for increasing physical activity.

Unfortunately, the influence of different types, amounts, and intensities of exercise has not been studied extensively in children. With respect to body fatness and exercise intensity, Bar-Or (103) recently concluded that there are too few data available to make a recommendation. In adults, Tremblay et al (104) found that high-intensity training was more effective in reducing body fatness than somewhat lower intensity training. If total energy used during the exercise sessions is the critical parameter, then simply lengthening the low-intensity sessions can allow the youth to use the same amount of energy as would be used in a high-intensity session. Savage et al (105) used this approach with prepubertal boys and found skinfold fat to decline similarly in the low- and high-intensity groups, even though the high-intensity training resulted in a clearer improvement in cardiovascular fitness. Even when the energy expenditure during the training itself is controlled, there are reasons to suspect that higher intensities may be more efficacious in reducing fatness if the intervention continues for a longer period than the typical 2–4 months seen in many exercise-only interventions. First, the exponential relationship between exercise intensity and postexercise metabolism may gradually lead to greater loss of fat as a result of high-intensity training. Secondly, if high-intensity training increases cardiovascular fitness more effectively, as shown by Savage et al (105), then the youth would be able progressively to use up more energy in a given amount of training time, eventually leading to greater fat loss. On the other hand, it may be that lower intensity exercise is more agreeable to obese children over the long term, resulting in greater adherence.

Outcomes of Family-Based Behavioral Interventions

The optimism associated with family-based behavioral interventions stems from evidence that this treatment approach may result in long-term benefits to obese children. Table 8-2 summarizes outcomes for family-based behavioral interventions reported at either 1, 5, or 10 years after initiating treatment. With the exception of the study by Israel et al (96), meaningful reductions in obesity status were a consistent finding at the 1-year mark. Of even greater interest are the 5-year results from the study by Johnson et al (94) and the combined 10-year results from the four studies of Epstein et al (106). These studies provide the most compelling evidence that the treatment of obesity in children can be successful over extended periods from childhood through adolescence to adulthood (102). From Epstein's perspective, two of the most helpful points to be distilled from their 10-year results are the recommendations that at least one parent be an active participant in the weight loss process, and that

Table 8-2 Outcomes for Family-based Behavioral Interventions for Childhood Obesity

Study	Year	Ages (yr)	n	Outcomes		
				1-year	5-year	10-year
Brownell et al (93)	1983	12–16	36	Percentage overweight: −10.7%; blood pressure: −1.9/−1.2 mmHg		
Mellin et al (100)	1987	12–18	34/29	Relative weight: −9.9% vs. −0.1% in control group		
Figueroa-Colon et al (98)	1993	7–17	7/4	Percentage overweight: −23% in protein-sparing diet group vs. −20% in hypocaloric diet group; blood pressure: −14/−15 mmHg when groups combined		

Israel et al (96)	1994	8–13	11/9	Percentage above triceps norm: +14.5% in enhanced treatment group vs. −1.8% in standard treatment group
Braet et al (99)	1997	7–16	60/49	Percentage overweight: −11% in experimental groups vs. +3.5% in control group
Johnson et al (94)	1997	8–16	12/6	Percentage of ideal body weight: −23% in experimental groups vs. −11% in control group
Epstein et al (106)	1994	6–12	158 (four studies)	30% of 158 children achieved non-obese status; 34% decreased percentage overweight by 20% or more

increasing physical activity is important for the maintenance of long-term weight control (92).

However, it has been noted that the 10-year follow-up studies were all conducted by the same North American research group and that there is need for other authors to replicate the research, particularly in a non-United States setting (107). Another observation is that the family-based behavioral intervention studies have tended to focus on outcomes related to simple anthropometric measurements such as percentage overweight or BMI. Left largely unexamined are the effects of these interventions on more direct measures of body fat and on the risk factors for obesity-related diseases such as CAD and NIDDM. It would be of considerable interest, for example, to know the effects of these interventions on fat patterning, especially visceral adipose tissue. In light of the relationship between visceral adipose tissue and CAD risk factors, it is important to clarify how training influences this fat depot. In a recent study of obese 7- to 11-year-olds, children who engaged in 4 months of after-school exercise without dietary intervention or behavior modification declined significantly in visceral fat as compared to the control group (108). Would this favorable result have been enhanced within the context of a long-term family-based behavioral intervention? Along the same lines, it would be important to know the extent to which a family-based behavioral intervention approach enhances the favorable results (reduced fatness and improved CAD risk factors) obtained in non-family-based interventions that utilized exercise alone (87), or diet plus exercise (109,110).

CONCLUSIONS

Childhood obesity is increasing in most modern societies, manifesting both short- and long-term deleterious consequences. The etiology of childhood obesity is complex, with genetic and environmental factors having contributory roles. However, there is reason to believe that the long-term treatment of childhood obesity can be successful. Family-based behavioral interventions, which integrate dietary change, increased physical activity, and behavior modification within a setting of family support, offer one pathway for achieving this success.

REFERENCES

1. Troiano RP, Flegal KM, Kuczmarski RJ, Campbell SM, Johnson CL. Overweight prevalence and trends for children and adolescents. National Health and Nutrition Examination Surveys, 1963–1991. Arch Pediatr Adolesc Med 1995; 149: 1085–1091.
2. Flegal KM. Defining obesity in children and adolescents: epidemiologic approaches. Crit Rev Food Sci Nutr 1993; 33: 307–312.
3. Power C, Lake JK, Cole TJ. Measurement and long-term health risks of child and adolescent fatness. Int J Obes Relat Metab Disord 1997; 21: 507–526.
4. Williams CL, Campanaro LA, Squillace M, Bollella M. Management of childhood obesity in pediatric practice. Ann N Y Acad Sci 1997; 817: 225–240.
5. Must A, Dallal GE, Dietz WH. Reference data for obesity: 85th and 95th percentiles of body mass index (wt/ht^2) and triceps skinfold thickness. Am J Clin Nutr 1991; 53: 839–846.
6. Williams DP, Going SB, Lohman TG, et al. Body fatness and risk for elevated blood pressure, total cholesterol, and serum lipoprotein ratios in children and adolescents. Am J Public Health 1992; 82: 358–363.
7. Himes JH, Dietz WH. Guidelines for overweight in adolescent preventive services: recommendations from an expert committee: Expert Committee on Clinical Guidelines for Overweight in Adolescent Preventive Services. Am J Clin Nutr 1994; 59: 307–316.
8. Gidding SS, Bao W, Srinivasan SR, Berenson GS. Effects of secular trends in obesity on coronary risk factors in children: the Bogalusa Heart Study. J Pediatr 1995; 127: 868–874.
9. Lehingue Y, Picot MC, Millot I, Fassio F. Increase in the prevalence of obesity among children aged 4–5 years in a French district between 1988 and 1993. Rev Epidemiol Sante Publique 1996; 44: 37–46 [in French].
10. Rona RJ. The National Study of Health and Growth (NSHG): 23 years on the road. Int J Epidemiol 1995; 24: S69–S74.

11. Berenson GS, Srinivasan SR, Bao W. Precursors of cardio-vascular risk in young adults from a biracial (black–white) population: the Bogalusa Heart Study. Ann N Y Acad Sci 1997; 817: 189–198.

12. Gutin B, Islam S, Manos T, Cucuzzo N, Smith C, Stachura ME. Relation of percentage of body fat and maximal aerobic capacity to risk factors for atherosclerosis and diabetes in black and white 7- to 11-year-old children. J Pediatr 1994; 125: 847–852.

13. Kikuchi DA, Srinivasan SR, Harsha DW, Webber LS, Sellers TA, Berenson GS. Relation of serum lipoprotein lipids and apolipoproteins to obesity in children: the Bogalusa Heart Study. Prev Med 1992; 21: 177–190.

14. Gutin B, Owens S, Treiber F, Islam S, Karp W, Slavens G. Weight-independent cardiovascular fitness and corónary risk factors. Arch Pediatr Adolesc Med 1997; 151: 462–465.

15. Lauer RM, Burns TL, Clarke WR, Mahoney LT. Childhood predictors of future blood pressure. Hypertension 1991; 18: 174–181.

16. McMurray RG, Harrel JS, Levine AA, Gansky SA. Childhood obesity elevates blood pressure and total cholesterol inde-pendent of physical activity. Int J Obes Relat Metab Disord 1995; 19: 881–886.

17. Reaven GM. Banting lecture 1988. Role of insulin resis-tance in human disease. Diabetes 1988; 37: 1595–1607.

18. Gutin B, Treiber F, Owens S, Mensah GA. Relations of body composition to left ventricular geometry and function in children. J Pediatr 1998; 132: 1023–1027.

19. Devereux RB, de Simone G, Ganau A, Roman MJ. Left ventricular hypertrophy and geometric remodeling in hypertension: stimuli, functional consequences and pro-gnostic implications. J Hypertens Suppl 1994; 12: 117–127.

20. de Simone G, Devereux RB, Mureddu GF, et al. Influence of obesity on left ventricular midwall mechanics in arterial hypertension. Hypertension 1996; 28: 276–283.

21. Treiber F, Papavassiliou D, Gutin B, et al. Determinants of endothelium-dependent femoral artery vasodilation in youth. Psychosom Med 1997; 59: 376–381.

22. Meredith IT, Anderson TJ, Uehata A, Yeung AC, Selwyn AP, Ganz P. Role of endothelium in ischemic coronary syn-dromes. Am J Cardiol 1993; 72: 27C–31C.

23. Celermajer DS. Endothelial dysfunction: does it matter? Is it reversible? J Am Coll Cardiol 1997; 30: 325–333.

24. Despres JP, Moorjani S, Ferland M, et al. Adipose tissue dis-tribution and plasma lipoprotein levels in obese women: importance of intra-abdominal fat. Arteriosclerosis 1989; 9: 203–210.

25. Pouliot MC, Despres JP, Nadeau A, et al. Visceral obesity in men: associations with glucose tolerance, plasma insulin, and lipoprotein levels. Diabetes 1992; 41: 826–834.

26. Rissanen J, Hudson R, Ross R. Visceral adiposity, androgens, and plasma lipids in obese men. Metabolism 1994; 43: 1318–1323.

27. Asayama K, Hayashibe H, Dobashi K, Uchida N, Kawada Y, Nakazawa S. Relationships between biochemical abnormalities and anthropometric indices of overweight, adiposity and body fat distribution in Japanese elementary school children. Int J Obes Relat Metab Disord 1995; 19: 253–259.

28. Daniels SR, Morrison JA, Sprecher DL, Khoury P, Kimball TR. Association of body fat distribution and cardiovascular risk factors in children and adolescents. Circulation 1999; 99: 541–545.

29. Goran MI, Kaskoun M, Shuman WP. Intra-abdominal adipose tissue in young children. Int J Obes Relat Metab Disord 1995; 19: 279–283.

30. Brambilla P, Manzoni P, Sironi S, et al. Peripheral and abdominal adiposity in childhood obesity. Int J Obes Relat Metab Disord 1994; 18: 795–800.

31. Caprio S, Hyman LD, McCarthy S, Lange R, Bronson M, Tamborlane WV. Fat distribution and cardiovascular risk factors in obese adolescent girls: importance of the intra-abdominal fat depot. Am J Clin Nutr 1996; 64: 12–17.

32. Yanovski JA, Yanovski SZ, Filmer KM, et al. Differences in body composition of black and white girls. Am J Clin Nutr 1996; 64: 833–839.

33. Braet C, Mervielde I, Vandereycken W. Psychological aspects of childhood obesity: a controlled study in a clinical and non-clinical sample. J Pediatr Psychol 1997; 22: 59–71.

34. Baum CG, Forehand R. Social factors associated with adolescent obesity. J Pediatr Psychol 1984; 9: 293–302.

35. Strauss CC, Smith K, Frame C, Forehand R. Personal and interpersonal characteristics associated with childhood obesity. J Pediatr Psychol 1985; 10: 337–343.

36. Richardson SA, Goodman N, Hastorf AH, et al. Cultural uniformity to physical disabilities. Am Sociol Rev 1961; 26: 241–247.

37. Maddox GL, Back KW, Liederman WR. Overweight as social deviance and disability. J Health Soc Behav 1968; 9: 287–298.

38. Bouchard C. Human variation in body mass: evidence for a role of the genes. Nutr Rev 1997; 55: S21–27; discussion S27–S30.

39. Miller WC, Lindeman AK, Wallace J, Niederpruem M. Diet composition, energy intake, and exercise in relation to body fat in men and women. Am J Clin Nutr 1990; 52: 426–430.

40. Segal KR, Gutin B. Thermic effects of food and exercise in lean and obese women. Metabolism 1983; 32: 581–589.

41. Davies PS, Wells JC, Fieldhouse CA, Day JM, Lucas A. Parental body composition and infant energy expenditure. Am J Clin Nutr 1995; 61: 1026–1029.

42. Schoeller DA, Bandini LG, Dietz WH. Inaccuracies in self-reported intake identified by comparison with the doubly labelled water method. Can J Physiol Pharmacol 1990; 68: 941–949.

43. Bandini LG, Schoeller DA, Cyr HN, Dietz WH. Validity of reported energy intake in obese and non-obese adolescents. Am J Clin Nutr 1990; 52: 421–425.

44. Briefel RR, McDowell MA, Alaimo K, et al. Total energy intake of the US population: the third National Health and Nutrition Examination Survey, 1988–1991. Am J Clin Nutr 1995; 62: 1072S–1080S.

45. Albertson AM, Tobelmann RC. Ten-year trend of energy intakes of American children ages 2–10 years. Ann N Y Acad Sci 1993; 699: 250–252.

46. Eck LH, Klesges RC, Hanson CL, Slawson D. Children at familial risk for obesity: an examination of dietary intake, physical activity and weight status. Int J Obes Relat Metab Disord 1992; 16: 71–78.

47. Nguyen VT, Larson DE, Johnson RK, Goran MI. Fat intake and adiposity in children of lean and obese parents. Am J Clin Nutr 1996; 63: 507–513.

48. Maffeis C, Pinelli L, Schutz Y. Fat intake and adiposity in 8- to 11-year-old obese children. Int J Obes Relat Metab Disord 1996; 20: 170–174.

49. Muecke L, Simons-Morton B, Huang IW, Parcel G. Is childhood obesity associated with high-fat foods and low physical activity? J Sch Health 1992; 62: 19–23.

50. Lissner L, Heitmann BL, Bengtsson C. Low-fat diets may prevent weight gain in sedentary women: prospective observations from the population study of women in Gothenburg, Sweden. Obes Res 1997; 5: 43–48.

51. Griffiths M, Payne PR. Energy expenditure in small children of obese and non-obese parents. Nature 1976; 260: 698–700.

52. Griffiths M, Payne PR, Stunkard AJ, Rivers JP, Cox M. Metabolic rate and physical development in children at risk of obesity. Lancet 1990; 336: 76–78.

53. Goran MI, Carpenter WH, McGloin A, Johnson R, Hardin JM, Weinsier RL. Energy expenditure in children of lean and obese parents. Am J Physiol 1995; 268: E917–E924.

54. Maffeis C, Schutz Y, Micciolo R, Zoccante L, Pinelli L. Resting metabolic rate in 6- to 10-year-old obese and non-obese children. J Pediatr 1993; 122: 556–562.

55. Fontvieille AM, Dwyer J, Ravussin E. Resting metabolic rate and body composition of Pima Indian and Caucasian children. Int J Obes Relat Metab Disord 1992; 16: 535–542.

56. Wells JC, Stanley M, Laidlaw AS, Day JM, Davies PS. The relationship between components of infant energy expenditure and childhood body fatness. Int J Obes Relat Metab Disord 1996; 20: 848–853.

57. Ravussin E, Swinburn BA. Pathophysiology of obesity. Lancet 1992; 340: 404–408.

58. Segal KR, Gutin B, Albu J, Pi-Sunyer FX. Thermic effects of food and exercise in lean and obese men of similar lean body mass. Am J Physiol 1987; 252: E110–E117.

59. Prentice AM, Goldberg GR, Murgatroyd PR, Cole TJ. Physical activity and obesity: problems in correcting expenditure for body size. Int J Obes Relat Metab Disord 1996; 20: 688–691.

60. Davies PS, Gregory J, White A. Physical activity and body fatness in pre-school children. Int J Obes Relat Metab Disord 1995; 19: 6–10.

61. Goran MI, Hunter G, Nagy TR, Johnson R. Physical activity related energy expenditure and fat mass in young children. Int J Obes Relat Metab Disord 1997; 21: 171–178.

62. Roberts SB, Savage J, Coward WA, Chew B, Lucas A. Energy expenditure and intake in infants born to lean and over-weight mothers. N Engl J Med 1988; 318: 461–466.

63. Deheeger M, Rolland-Cachera MF, Fontvieille AM. Physical activity and body composition in 10-year-old French children: linkages with nutritional intake? Int J Obes Relat Metab Disord 1997; 21: 372–379.

64. Mo-suwan L, Geater AF. Risk factors for childhood obesity in a transitional society in Thailand. Int J Obes Relat Metab Disord 1996; 20: 697–703.

65. Klesges RC, Klesges LM, Eck LH, Shelton ML. A longitudinal analysis of accelerated weight gain in preschool children. Pediatrics 1995; 95: 126–130.

66. Moore LL, Nguyen US, Rothman KJ, Cupples LA, Ellison RC. Preschool physical activity level and change in body fatness in young children: the Framingham Children's Study. Am J Epidemiol 1995; 142: 982–988.

67. Gortmaker SL, Must A, Sobol AM, Peterson K, Colditz GA, Dietz WH. Television viewing as a cause of increasing obesity among children in the United States, 1986–1990. Arch Pediatr Adolesc Med 1996; 150: 356–362.

68. Crespo CJ, Smit E, Troiano RP, Bartlett SJ, Macera CA, Andersen RE. Television watching, energy intake, and obesity in US children: results from the third National Health and Nutrition Examination Survey, 1988–1994. Arch Pediatr Adolesc Med 2001; 155: 360–365.

69. DuRant RH, Baranowski T, Johnson M, Thompson WO. The relationship among television watching, physical activity, and body composition of young children. Pediatrics 1994; 94: 449–455.

70. Goran MI. Metabolic precursors and effects of obesity in children: a decade of progress, 1990–1999. Am J Clin Nutr 2001; 73: 158–171.

71. Janz KF, Mahoney LT. Three-year follow-up of changes in aerobic fitness during puberty: the Muscatine Study. Res Q Exerc Sport 1997; 68: 1–9.

72. Johnson MS, Figueroa-Colon R, Herd SL, et al. Aerobic fitness, not energy expenditure, influences subsequent increase in adiposity in black and white children. Pediatrics 2000; 106: E50.

73. Tremblay A, Despres JP, Leblanc C, et al. Effect of intensity of physical activity on body fatness and fat distribution. Am J Clin Nutr 1990; 51: 153–157.

74. Mayers N, Gutin B. Physiological characteristics of elite pre-pubertal cross-country runners. Med Sci Sports 1979; 11: 172–176.

75. Saris WH. Effects of energy restriction and exercise on the sympathetic nervous system. Int J Obes Relat Metab Disord 1995; 19 (suppl 7): 17–23.

76. Zurlo F, Ferraro RT, Fontvielle AM, Rising R, Bogardus C, Ravussin E. Spontaneous physical activity and obesity: cross-sectional and longitudinal studies in Pima Indians. Am J Physiol 1992; 263: E296–E300.

77. Caprio S, Tamborlane WV, Silver D, et al. Hyperleptinemia: an early sign of juvenile obesity—relations to body fat depots and insulin concentrations. Am J Physiol 1996; 271: E626–E630.

78. Lahlou N, Landais P, De Boissieu D, Bougneres PF. Circulating leptin in normal children and during the dynamic phase of juvenile obesity: relation to body fatness, energy metabolism, caloric intake, and sexual dimorphism. Diabetes 1997; 46: 989–993.

79. Salbe AD, Nicolson M, Ravussin E. Total energy expenditure and the level of physical activity correlate with plasma leptin concentrations in 5-year-old children. J Clin Invest 1997; 99: 592–595.

80. Nagy TR, Gower BA, Trowbridge CA, Dezenberg C, Shewchuk RM, Goran MI. Effects of gender, ethnicity, body composition, and fat distribution on serum leptin concentrations

in children. J Clin Endocrinol Metab 1997; 82: 2148–2152.

81. Williamson DF, Madans J, Anda RF, Kleinman JC, Kahn HS, Byers T. Recreational physical activity and 10-year weight change in a US national cohort. Int J Obes Relat Metab Disord 1993; 17: 279–286.

82. Bouchard C. Obesity in adulthood: the importance of childhood and parental obesity. N Engl J Med 1997; 337: 926–927.

83. Whitaker RC, Wright JA, Pepe MS, Seidel KD, Dietz WH. Predicting obesity in young adulthood from childhood and parental obesity. N Engl J Med 1997; 337: 869–873.

84. Maffeis C, Schutz Y, Pinelli L. Effect of weight loss on resting energy expenditure in obese prepubertal children. Int J Obes Relat Metab Disord 1992; 16: 41–47.

85. Schwingshandl J, Borkenstein M. Changes in lean body mass in obese children during a weight reduction program: effect on short term and long term outcome. Int J Obes Relat Metab Disord 1995; 19: 752–755.

86. Ballor DL, Poehlman ET. Exercise-training enhances fat-free mass preservation during diet-induced weight loss: a meta-analytical finding. Int J Obes Relat Metab Disord 1994; 18: 35–40.

87. Sasaki J, Shindo M, Tanaka H, Ando M, Arakawa K. A long-term aerobic exercise program decreases the obesity index and increases the high density lipoprotein cholesterol concentration in obese children. Int J Obes 1987; 11: 339–345.

88. Blomquist B, Borjeson M, Larsson Y, Persson B, Sterky G. The effect of physical activity on the body measurements and work capacity of overweight boys. Acta Paediatr Scand 1965; 54: 566–572.

89. Seltzer CC, Mayer J. An effective weight control program in a public school system. Am J Public Health Nations Health 1970; 60: 679–689.

90. Gutin B, Cucuzzo N, Islam S, Smith C, Moffatt R, Pargman D. Physical training improves body composition of black obese 7- to 11-year-old girls. Obes Res 1995; 3: 305–312.

91. Gutin B, Owens S, Riggs S, et al. Effect of physical training on cardiovascular health in obese children. In: Armstrong N, Kirby B, Welsman J, eds. XIXth International Symposium of the European Group of Pediatric Work Physiology. University of Exeter, UK: E & FN Spon, London, 1997: 382–389.

92. Epstein LH. Family-based behavioural intervention for obese children. Int J Obes Relat Metab Disord 1996; 20 (suppl 1): 14–21.

93. Brownell KD, Kelman JH, Stunkard AJ. Treatment of obese

children with and without their mothers: changes in weight and blood pressure. Pediatrics 1983; 71: 515–523.

94. Johnson WG, Hinkle LK, Carr RE, et al. Dietary and exercise interventions for juvenile obesity: long-term effect of behavioral and public health models. Obes Res 1997; 5: 257–261.

95. Epstein LH, Wing RR, Koeske R, Andrasik F, Ossip DJ. Child and parent weight loss in family-based behavior modification programs. J Consult Clin Psychol 1981; 49: 674–685.

96. Israel AC, Guile CA, Baker JE, Silverman WK. An evaluation of enhanced self-regulation training in the treatment of childhood obesity. J Pediatr Psychol 1994; 19: 737–749.

97. Epstein LH, Valoski AM, Vara LS, et al. Effects of decreasing sedentary behavior and increasing activity on weight change in obese children. Health Psychol 1995; 14: 109–115.

98. Figueroa-Colon R, von Almen TK, Franklin FA, Schuftan C, Suskind RM. Comparison of two hypocaloric diets in obese children. Am J Dis Child 1993; 147: 160–166.

99. Braet C, Van Winckel M, Van Leeuwen K. Follow-up results of different treatment programs for obese children. Acta Paediatr 1997; 86: 397–402.

100. Mellin LM, Slinkard LA, Irwin CE, Jr. Adolescent obesity intervention: validation of the SHAPEDOWN program. J Am Diet Assoc 1987; 87: 333–338.

101. Dietz WH. Therapeutic strategies in childhood obesity. Horm Res 1993; 39: 86–90.

102. Gill TP. Key issues in the prevention of obesity. Br Med Bull 1997; 53: 359–388.

103. Bar-Or O, Baranowski T. Physical activity, adiposity, and obesity among adolescents. Pediatr Exerc Sci 1994; 6: 348–360.

104. Tremblay A, Simoneau JA, Bouchard C. Impact of exercise intensity on body fatness and skeletal muscle metabolism. Metabolism 1994; 43: 814–818.

105. Savage MP, Petratis MM, Thomson WH, Berg K, Smith JL, Sady SP. Exercise training effects on serum lipids of prepubescent boys and adult men. Med Sci Sports Exerc 1986; 18: 197–204.

106. Epstein LH, Valoski A, Wing RR, McCurley J. Ten-year outcomes of behavioral family-based treatment for childhood obesity. Health Psychol 1994; 13: 373–383.

107. Glenny AM, O'Meara S, Melville A, Sheldon TA, Wilson C. The treatment and prevention of obesity: a systematic review of the literature. Int J Obes Relat Metab Disord 1997; 21: 715–737.

108. Owens S, Gutin B, Allison J, et al. Effect of physical training on total and visceral fat in obese children. Med Sci Sports Exerc 1999; 31: 143–148.

109. Becque MD, Katch VL, Rocchini AP, Marks CR, Moorehead C. Coronary risk incidence of obese adolescents: reduction by exercise plus diet intervention. Pediatrics 1988; 81: 605–612.
110. Rocchini AP, Katch V, Schork A, Kelch RP. Insulin and blood pressure during weight loss in obese adolescents. Hypertension 1987; 10: 267–273.

Chapter 9

Obesity and Health: Public Policy Implications and Recommendations

Kathleen J. Melanson, Kyle J. McInnis, and James M. Rippe

The World Health Organization has described the escalating global obesity epidemic as one of the greatest neglected public health problems of our time, with an impact on health that may well prove to be as great as that of smoking (1). The United States government, in its 1995 Dietary Guidelines for Americans, listed obesity as one of the major nutrition-related health problems facing the nation (2). According to data from the Centers for Disease Control and Prevention (CDC), the prevalence and severity of obesity has increased rapidly since then (3), with no parts of the population spared, and no signs of abating (3). The rise of obesity in US men and women from 1998 to 1999 is depicted in Figure 9-1.

This new century brings growing challenges and opportunities for health professionals who assist individuals in body weight management, as well as for scientists seeking to advance knowledge regarding obesity, energy balance regulation, and optimal health. Although obesity is a chronic condition, it is spreading with the speed and dispersion characteristic of a communicable disease epidemic (1,3–5). With the escalating obesity epidemic negatively impacting multi-

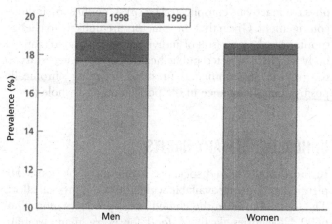

Figure 9-1 Increase in obesity prevalence among adults, by gender, 1998–99. (From Mokdad et al (3).)

ple chronic diseases (6,7) (see also Chapter 7), economic burdens (8), and quality of life (9,10), heightened efforts are crucial from clinical, scientific and, more so than ever, public health standpoints.

As with most public health issues, curtailing the rise in obesity must involve a systematic approach. This includes explicating the problem and its causes, identifying optimal yet realistic goals, determining the most efficacious and efficient means of working toward those goals, developing guidelines and concrete strategies, integrating and implementing the guidelines and strategies, and assessing ongoing outcomes (11,12). In the case of obesity, solutions are necessarily multifaceted, because of the heterogeneity of the etiology of obesity. Although genetic predisposition doubtlessly contributes to the accretion of excess adiposity, heritable factors cannot account for the mounting prevalence and severity of obesity in recent decades (13). Furthermore, genetic factors are less subject to control by clinical and public health measures than are the lifestyle factors that are the critical underpinnings of the obesity epidemic. The central lifestyle factors involve unhealthy dietary habits and physical inactivity, complicated by stress, confusion, and discouragement. Given that these factors are unlikely to change spontaneously as a result of individual motivation to manage body weight, concerted public health efforts are necessary to reverse the environmental pressures fostering chronically positive energy balance in the population as a whole (5).

UNHEALTHY DIETARY HABITS

In most industrialized societies, highly palatable foods are plentiful and readily available with little or no physical effort. The food industry in the United States produces more than 6600 kilocalories (kcal) of food for every man, woman, and child in the country every day (14). Between 1970 and 1994, per capita energy availability increased by 15.2%, and fat availability increased 21.8% according to estimates from the US Department of Agriculture, US Food Supply Service (14). Americans spend, on average, 38–50% of their food dollars on meals prepared outside the home, with the most frequently ordered item being hamburgers (14–16). Frequency of restaurant food consumption has been positively correlated with dietary energy and fat intake (17), and with body fatness (18). Although nearly three fourths of American adults consume fat-reduced products (19), they are likely to be consuming them in larger portions (20,21). The number and magnitude of super-size portions offered on menus and in stores has been increasing steadily in response to consumer demand (22–25). The enormous quantity and variety of food, which is typically high-fat, energy-dense, palatable, and easily accessible, is advertised with billions of dollars. For example, the annual promotion budget for McDonald's food chain is over 1 billion dollars (26), as compared to that for the National Cancer Institute's "5-A-Day" fruit and vegetable campaign (27), which is 1 million dollars.

Data from several sources, including the third National Health and Nutrition Examination Survey (NHANES III), suggest upward trends in total daily energy intake of Americans in recent years (20,28–30). Much of this increase was likely caused by energy-dense nutrient-poor foods such as sweetened beverages, desserts, snacks, fats, and sweeteners (31,32). The amount and variety of energy-dense nutrient-poor foods produced in the United States has increased at significantly greater rates than that of fruit and vegetable availability (33). An estimated one third of the population consumes an average of 45% of daily energy from foods classified as energy-dense nutrient-poor (31). Not only does consumption of high-fat highly refined foods and low consumption of fruits, vegetables, and whole grains predispose to many chronic diseases such as cardiovascular diseases and cancer, but energy overconsumption is believed to be instrumental in the increasing prevalence and severity of obesity (21,31,32,34). Dietary factors are associated with five of the 10 leading causes of death in the United States; over 30% of national health care expenditures is related to inappropriate diet (35).

PHYSICAL INACTIVITY

Compounding the overconsumption of energy-dense foods and beverages is the prevalence of sedentary lifestyle behaviors. Use of computers, automobiles, power-driven lawn mowers, elevators, and other time- and energy-saving devices, along with sedentary leisure time activities such as television and video games, has become the norm, contributing to further reduction in physical activity and energy expenditure. In many urban and suburban communities, fear of danger often discourages people from walking or recreating outdoors (36). Often, neighborhoods are structured so that getting to stores or other central areas in a reasonable amount of time requires automotive transport (12,36). Furthermore, many school districts have reduced or eliminated physical education and sports programs, and other opportunities for students to be active during the day (34). Although participation in leisure time physical activity in the population as a whole has remained steady, it averages below levels required to maintain health, and most data indicate that energy expended in daily lifestyle physical activities has dropped while sedentary behaviors have increased (21).

An estimated 24% of the United States' population accumulates the minimum recommended level of moderate physical activity daily, 52% are intermittently active, and 25% are entirely sedentary (37). A sedentary lifestyle contributes to many health conditions independent of body weight. Additionally, this inactive trend has played a major part in the chronically positive energy balance leading to the surge of obesity in industrialized countries (21).

STRESS

Life in technologically advanced societies is becoming increasingly more complicated, stressful, and fast-paced, which may also indirectly contribute to the rise in obesity. Many individuals blame tight schedules for permitting little time for physical activity, and promoting consumption of fast food or convenience foods. Mounting evidence suggests that individuals are overeating in response to stress, anxiety, or other negative emotions at greater rates than ever (38). Eating is often a coping or escape mechanism for many people (39) and, in these cases, food may be seen as an abused substance (40). According to some investigators and clinicians, overeating may become an addictive behavior (38).

CONFUSION AND DISCOURAGEMENT

The majority of obese individuals express concern about the health implications of their weight; however, inaccurate information and discouragement regarding weight management abound (41). Nearly half of US women, and more than one third of US men report that they are attempting to lose weight (42). The general public is constantly being fed misinformation about solutions to weight control, which leads to prevalent confusion and unhealthful self-initiated approaches to weight loss. The proliferation of misinformation about magic solutions to weight loss is apparent through newspapers, magazines, television, and websites. Consumers are led to believe that quick and easy remedies can be purchased to cure obesity, when the truth is that the only way to keep off excess weight is through lifelong behaviors involving physical activity, balanced with a healthy diet. When individuals repeatedly attempt the magical solutions promoted through much of the media, and are repeatedly met with failure, they become increasingly discouraged (43).

SPECIAL POPULATIONS TO CONSIDER

Lower Socioeconomic Status

Lower educational levels and socioeconomic status (SES) are associated with higher obesity rates, less health knowledge, and lower participation in physical activity (3,4,44). Increases in obesity prevalence from 1998 to 1999 in US adults according to educational levels are shown in Figure 9-2 (3). Low SES has been shown to correlate with more rapid rates of adult weight gain relative to higher SES, with an inverse correlation between SES and body mass index (BMI) increases (45). Health-related quality of life has been shown to correlate positively with SES, which was partly explained

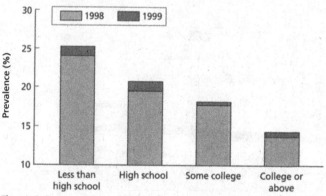

Figure 9-2 Increase in obesity prevalence among adults, by educational level, 1998–99. (From Mokdad et al (3).)

by self-efficacy, suggesting that enhancing self-efficacy in low SES groups may be an important component of health promotion in this segment of the population (46). Inequitable access to health education, treatment services, and environmental opportunities for healthful lifestyle behaviors, as well as social or cultural practices, beliefs or attitudes, may be responsible for the exacerbation of obesity and its comorbidities in lower socioeconomic groups (12,47).

Racial Ethnic Minorities

Minority populations, especially minority women, are at greatest risk for obesity, and hence its comorbidities (48). According to data from the CDC, the obesity prevalence in whites, Hispanics, and black people is 17.7, 21.5, and 27.3%, respectively (3). Nearly 50% of African American and Mexican women are obese, with prevalences of 60 and 70%, respectively, for the age range of 45–55 years for women in these racial ethnic groups (49). From 1991 to 1998, the prevalence of obesity among Hispanic Americans rose by 80%, and among black people by 39.2% (5). However, these are the first data indicating that the increase in obesity prevalence was greater for white (47.3%) than for black people (39.2%). Recent increases in different racial ethnic groups are shown graphically in Figure 9-3 (3).

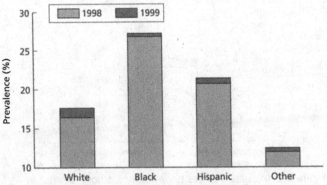

Figure 9-3 Increase in obesity prevalence among adults, by race/ethnicity, 1998–99. (From Mokdad et al (3).)

Children

The number of children in the United States who are overweight has more than doubled in the last decade (50). More than 10% of children age 4–5 years are obese, as are 21% of 12- to 19-years-olds (49), the highest levels in United States history. It is highly likely that children and adolescents in modern societies are at risk for obesity, because their lifestyles are more sedentary than those of previous generations. One fourth of United States children watch, on average, ≥4 h/day of television (51), and approximately 44% of children have a television in their bedroom (52). The average child views 10,000 food commercials each year, with 95% of these being for candy, fast food, soft drinks, and sugared cereals (38). It has been estimated that as much as 50% of children's energy intake comes from energy-dense nutrient-poor foods while they fail to meet the recommended daily servings of fruit, vegetables, and dairy (51,53). Soft drink energy consumption has been shown to be significantly higher in overweight than in lean children (54).

Multiple cardiovascular risk factors have been identified in large proportions of overweight school-age children (55). These children and adolescents are highly predisposed to hypercholesterolemia, glucose intolerance, and other risk factors that are very likely to carry over into adulthood chronic diseases (6,55–57). Adolescents who are obese experience discrimination on a variety of levels: they enter the job market at lower salaries than do peers who are not obese, and may never recover from this economic disadvantage (58,59). Therefore, with the rising prevalence, severity, and comorbidities of obesity in children and adolescents, the population is storing up health, and possibly economic, problems for the future (see also Chapter 8).

The Aging Population

The age composition of the United States' population has changed dramatically during the 20th century as the baby boomer generation enters the fifth, sixth and seventh decades of life, and as life expectancy increases. By the end of the 1990s, one in every four persons was aged 50 years and over. It is estimated that by the year 2030, the proportion of the population in this age category will be about one in three (60). For the first time in US history, the national census forms had three digits for age, to accommodate the 70,000 centenarians in the country (61). The expanding older population is of concern because weight tends to increase with advancing age, starting as early as the midtwenties, carrying obesity-related chronic disease risk with it (62). The percentage of obese adults declines among the most elderly, but visceral adiposity may still increase, particularly among postmenopausal women (3,62,63). Of all age groups, the range from 40 to 69 years has the highest prevalence of obesity (21–24%) (3). In the 50–59 year age group, obesity increased 48% from 1991 to 1998 (5). Heavier weight in middle age has been associated with greater cardiovascular risk and mobility problems in older age (63). Therefore, prevention of weight gain and obesity during mid-life may assure healthier elder years.

ECONOMIC BURDENS

The direct and indirect costs of obesity to individuals and to society have been increasing along with the rise in the prevalence and severity of obesity. In addition to the >$30 billion spent each year in the United States on weight loss treatments and diet products (most of which offer no demonstrable long-term success), an estimated $68 billion is spent on clinical complications directly related to obesity, including diabetes, hypertension, osteoarthritis, and cardiovascular diseases (7,8). An estimated 5.7% of annual United States' health care costs (in 1995 dollars) and lost productivity are directly caused by obesity. When indirect costs are factored in, this estimate may be as high as 10% (4). From 1988 to 1994, the number of physician visits attributable to obesity-related conditions increased by 88% (8). Approximately 52.6 million sick days are lost each year because of illnesses and disabilities directly related to obesity and inactivity (64). More than $22 billion is spent each year on health care costs related to the cardiovascular complications of obesity (65).

"HEALTHY PEOPLE GOALS"

In recent years, progress has been made in identifying factors involved in the development of obesity, and guidelines aimed at avoiding this development. However, there has been an apparent lag in translation of such progress into action and monitoring implementation in order to develop corrective measures at the operational level.

In 1990, the CDC established a comprehensive set of 315 preventive health objectives toward making the nation healthier by the year 2000. Of these "Healthy People 2000 Goals", only 15% were achieved, 44% progressed, and 18% worsened (66). Among the goals that moved in a negative direction relative to the objectives were overweight and physical inactivity, with increases rather than decreases in both of these, as compared to the 1990 baseline levels. At the outset of this new century, 467 new objectives have been set in the "Healthy People 2010 Goals". The two main objectives of this document are to increase the number of years of healthy life and to eliminate racial and ethnic health disparities. Among the 10 major health indicators identified to serve as the nation's heath report card in this document, the first two listed are physical activity, and overweight and obesity (67). The indicators summarize the numerous goals into tangible outcomes, to prevent the public from becoming overwhelmed, and can be used to develop specific action plans at various levels, and to track progress. For all health care professionals, the intention is not only to focus on the goals of Healthy People 2010, but to work proactively to ensure that positive strides are made toward achieving them. It will be a major challenge to reverse the trends that evaded the Healthy People 2000 goals, particularly for the obesity epidemic, but continued advancement and application of knowledge about obesity prevention and treatment is urgently needed, and health professionals must work

Table 9-1 Summary of Healthy People 2010 Goals Related to Overweight and Obesity	
Goal	Increase the proportion of adults who are at a healthy weight
Target	60%
Baseline	42% of adults age ≥20 years had BMI = 18.5–25.0 in 1988–94
Goal	Reduce the proportion of adults who are obese
Target	15%
Baseline	23% of adults age ≥20 years had BMI ≥30 in 1988–94
Goal	Reduce the proportion of children and adolescents who are overweight or obese
Targets	5% for all age groups
Baseline	10–11% for children and adolescents age 6–19 years

together to progress toward the goals. The Healthy People 2010 Goals for Overweight and Obesity are summarized in Table 9-1.

REVERSING THE CAUSES OF THE OBESITY EPIDEMIC

Advances in molecular biology have elucidated numerous genetic links to obesity (68). However, the explosion of prevalence and severity of obesity in the past several decades cannot be attributable solely to genes, because it is unlikely that the gene pool has changed so dramatically within this period (13). Genetic predisposition to obesity may render one susceptible to accretion of excess body weight, but an environment promoting sedentary behavior and excess energy and fat intake, driven by non-salubrious behaviors and attitudes ultimately determines whether one becomes obese (69). The prevailing trend of individuals turning to weight loss gimmicks, fads, and remedies must be turned into a trend of increased participation in daily physical activity and more healthful dietary habits.

A challenging yet critical undertaking for both scientists and policy makers will be integrating scientific knowledge and policy formation (35). Public health messages must focus increasingly on balancing energy intake and expenditure (5,36). Fundamental changes must be made in areas currently lacking efforts to control the obesity epidemic. Modification of governmental policies and programs offers great potential for changing current environmental forces promoting poor diet and sedentary behavior. For example, current regulations governing communities, workplaces, schools, medical centers and other venues could be modified to make the environments more conducive to healthful diet and physical activity patterns (34). Furthermore, government regulation of education, mass media, food labeling and advertising, food assistance, health care and training, transportation, and urban development has potential for influencing the environment in such a way to promote healthier lifestyles (11,12).

Policies to improve health and reduce obesity must encompass nutrition and exercise objectives within economic growth and development, agriculture, food production and processing, marketing, environmental management, health care, education, and research. Educational methods must be improved to better inform and motivate consumers about health, to encourage food producers and manufacturers to supply healthier foods, to urge community leaders to develop better areas for physical activity, to ensure training of future professionals, and to provide legislators with the basis to make informed decisions (11,12,34–36). Additionally, the mass media has a particularly strong influence on a society's beliefs, values, practices, and trends. Therefore, this sector should also become informed and involved, to promote more positive attitudes towards health, food, and physical activity (12).

PREVENTION

The optimal goal regarding the obesity epidemic is a decline in the prevalence and severity of excess weight in all age, ethnic, socioeconomic, and geographic groups. Over the past several decades, public health efforts to prevent the rise of obesity have failed, affirming that to actually reverse the trend is a formidable undertaking. Therefore, the most appropriate focus at present may be prevention, aiming to halt the rise in the prevalence and severity of obesity before attempting to cause a downward trend in the nation's BMI. While treatments to reverse obesity must actively involve physicians and other health care professionals, prevention of obesity must start at the population level (41). National leadership is needed to ensure the participation of health officials and researchers, educators and legislators, transportation experts and urban planners, food industries and restaurants, the mass media, businesses, community organizations, and non-profit groups, all working together to formulate a public health campaign with a better chance of success (34). Research on obesity prevention is limited, and urgently needed, as is a sustained plan of action (38). A national comprehensive obesity prevention strategy must be developed to incorporate educational, behavioral, and environmental components.

Increases in BMI have occurred across the full range of weight-for-height categories in the population. However, increases are most marked at the upper end of the BMI distribution, with the heaviest people becoming heavier (70). This suggests that individuals who are already obese may be most susceptible to the environmental forces that promote weight gain. Therefore, prevention efforts must include a focus on the avoidance of weight gain among those who are already obese, in addition to preventing the development of obesity in those who are not currently obese. This need for prevention is reinforced by data demonstrating that weight gain itself is a risk factor for the development of chronic diseases (see Chapter 7).

Federal, state, local, and private sector involvement is called for in preventing the ongoing rise in the obesity epidemic. The food industry can have a role in obesity prevention by increasing availability of healthful products that are convenient, affordable and appealing, served in reasonable portion sizes, and appropriately labeled (34,35). Restaurants and other vendors of meals and snacks prepared outside the home can provide nutrition information on menus or wrappers (34). They can also play a part in advocating healthful foods and diets, recognizing that it is overall diet, physical activity, and lifestyle that matters. They can communicate health-related messages and help to educate the public. For example, some cereal boxes have information on their back panel regarding tips for improving lifestyle and health. The Food and Drug Administration (FDA) has approved several health claims for package labeling. The food industry can partner with organizations at multiple levels to support initiatives, education, resources, and research to promote healthy weight management (11).

Increasing healthful food and beverage selections should become a priority for schools, workplaces, community facilities, and other public places. Purchases of fruits and vegetables from cafeterias and vending machines have been shown to double when their prices were cut in half (71). Therefore, a strategy whereby healthful foods are made less costly, while energy-dense nutrient-poor foods are made more costly, may be effective in promoting more healthful food purchases (72). Although resistance to this strategy may be met from the food and beverage industry, the health of the nation is more critical than private or commercial sector interests, and such strategies may encourage these industries to produce more healthful foods and beverages.

Enhancing the level of physical activity of the population must involve efforts at various levels, including education regarding the health benefits of exercise independent of body weight, increased access to places for physical activity such as walking and bike paths, parks, gyms, public swimming pools and skating rinks, pedestrian-only zones in urban shopping areas, availability of community physical activity programs and organized sports, community infrastructure that fosters more frequent walks or bike rides for errands, less dependence on motorized transport, and increased opportunities to be physically active at school and work (12,34,36).

Decreases in BMI, triceps skinfold thickness, and waist circumference over 7 months have been reported in children who decreased the number of hours spent watching television or playing video games as compared to controls (52). Not only may the sedentary behavior and lack of physical activity that occurs with television and video game use be instrumental in the development of obesity, but eating snack foods and meals in front of the television, and viewing advertisements for candy, fast foods, and soft drinks may be promoting positive energy balance as well (34). Thus, an effective strategy to help reverse childhood obesity may be to increase children's opportunities for, and awareness of, physically active behaviors to replace sedentary behaviors such as television viewing and video game playing. The importance of physical education in schools cannot be overstated. Particularly problematic are the declines in the number of students receiving physical education, the lack of time dedicated for these classes, and the way existing classes are taught (34,36). Studies have shown that most students are only active an average of 5 min during a 1-h physical education class (37). Because few opportunities exist to be physically active after school, school time must be used to accumulate periods of physical activity. The emphasis must be on activities that are perceived to be most enjoyable for the children, as is also the case for adults.

POTENTIAL MODELS

In undertaking a major public health strategy to overcome the obesity epidemic, it may prove useful to consider existing approaches that have successfully mitigated other significant health problems. The decline in tobacco use resulted from concerted efforts at various levels, including national advertising campaigns to increase awareness of the health hazards of smoking, smoke-free policies in public places, taxes on cigarettes, and warnings on labels (36). Although inducing a decline in the prevalence and severity of obesity should also involve concerted efforts at various levels, some fundamental differences exist in the approach to obesity.

People cannot, and should not, entirely stop eating in the same way as they can quit smoking; rather, they must improve their dietary choices and habits while increasing daily energy expenditure. This involves detailed educational efforts and materials on making appropriate selections in an environment abundant with energy-dense nutrient-poor snacks, fast food, processed foods, desserts, and beverages, as well as prevailing opportunities for sedentary behavior over physical activity. It will also require increasing the availability of affordable fruits, vegetables, whole grains, and lean sources of protein in restaurants, workplaces, schools, vending machines, and other social situations, as well as promoting positive attitudes and possibilities for daily physical activity. People cannot "just say no" to eating, as was promoted to "just say no" to drugs. However, they can "just say no" to junk food, and "just say yes" to exercise, although putting these statements into practice will entail major changes in attitudes toward lifestyle behaviors. Balance, moderation, and awareness are key elements. The challenge lies in effectively integrating these principles into societies where excess is the norm.

Over the past century, medical science has virtually eradicated many serious diseases such as polio, tuberculosis, and measles. During this time, life expectancy has increased from 45 to 75 years (61). In the relatively young science of nutrition, many nutritional problems have been overcome or minimized, including rickets, scurvy, pellagra, goiter, and dental caries. These achievements were accomplished through intensive research and evidence-based action. In the advent of this new century, one of the most serious health problems facing much of the industrialized world is the obesity epidemic, which at this point seems out of control. A similar tactic of systematic research and multifaceted action will be most appropriate for overcoming obesity, but with essential modifications. Preventing and managing obesity involves efforts to resist or reverse a positive energy balance through a combination of increased energy expenditure and decreased energy intake (21). Many factors influence this balance, including genetic, environmental, and behavioral which must all be taken into account. Furthermore, body weight can be a personal sensitive issue, and attitudes regarding body size and shape are strongly influenced by social, cultural, and personal factors. Thus, it is critical that efforts to reverse the obesity epidemic do not stigmatize obese individuals. The approach must be non-judgmental and focused on health outcomes rather than on body weight (38). Everyone wants to be healthy. By concentrating on improving health outcomes rather than weight, the focus on the aesthetic aspects can be avoided, as well as possible perceptions of discrimination against obese individuals. As stated by Koplan and Dietz (36), "Implementation of such strategies will require a shift in emphasis from a cosmetic ideal weight for height to an acceptable weight for health." As endeavors are made to reverse the obesity epidemic, health professionals should envision the turn of the next century, when advances in medicine and health will be historically viewed, and they look back and comment that the obesity epidemic was a thing of the past.

Other extensive programs that have been effective in addressing chronic diseases include the National Diabetes Education Program, National Cholesterol Education Program, and National High Blood Pressure Education Program. A similar program for obesity education would be highly appropriate. Advancement toward necessary policy implementation aimed at obesity prevention can be anticipated through the publication of the first Surgeon General's Report on Obesity, in January 2002 (34).

FUTURE DIRECTIONS

Leaders in the health care, scientific, public policy, and educational professions must be proactive in raising public consciousness of lifestyle behaviors that promote healthy weight. Concerted efforts from these professions can provide substantial preventive, educational, and treatment programs for people of all ages and socioeconomic groups. Some possible actions for each of these areas are listed in this section. Specific recommendations for various groups involved in reducing the public health problem of obesity are listed in Table 9-2.

Table 9-2 Recommendations for Groups Involved in Reducing the Public Health Problem of Obesity

MEDICAL PROFESSIONALS
- Routinely assess BMI and waist circumference to monitor temporal changes
- Counsel patients on the health benefits of avoiding weight gain
- Educate overweight/obese patients on health benefits of modest weight loss
- Become educated, and educate on techniques for safe effective weight loss
- Attend continuing education programs relating to obesity management
- Integrate dietitians, exercise physiologists, nurses, and behaviorists into multidisciplinary treatment approaches
- Stay in tune with, or participate in, current obesity research

HEALTH CARE SERVICES
- Provide appropriate coverage for obesity treatment by physicians, dietitians, exercise physiologists, behaviorists, etc.
- Provide incentives for the service provider physician networks to work toward obesity prevention and thereby risk reduction
- Provide educational materials for member-patients to inform them of the health risks of obesity
- Increase availability of options for referrals for obesity treatment

EMPLOYERS
- Work with insurers, medical institutions, and others to develop healthy lifestyle programs that emphasize reduction or prevention of obesity
- Encourage consumption of healthful cafeteria foods and participation in readily available exercise programs within the workplace
- Distribute materials on healthy lifestyle options that can be realistically incorporated into daily living

Table 9-2 continues

Table 9-2 (*Continued*)

- Ensure that employees have medical insurance coverage for health care services related to healthy weight management

GOVERNMENT
- Establish a National Obesity Education Program prioritizing prevention and treatment, along with the Surgeon General's Report on Obesity
- Amend Medicare and Medicaid to assure that obesity assessment and management is available to elderly, disabled, and all socioeconomic classes
- Provide culturally sensitive client education materials for use by welfare, social service systems, and other government agencies
- Encourage state medical associations to require completion of nutrition and exercise physiology courses for obtaining and retaining licenses
- Encourage food manufacturers to use marketing to develop and promote more nutritious and less energy-dense food choices
- Promote more healthful cafeteria food selections in schools and worksites
- Educate children to make healthful food choices and become more active
- Increase Physical Education and Health Education requirements and participation in public schools
- Reward participation in physical activities in schools and worksites
- Encourage state and local municipalities to expand the role of public health departments to collaborate with schools, service providers, and employers in the development and implementation of public education programs aimed at reducing obesity and increasing physical activity
- Promote an environment and community resources that favor increased physical activity and salubrious diet (walking and bike paths, public swimming pools, skating rinks, safe areas for recreation, sports programs, healthy food choices in restaurants and cafeterias, health-promoting programs in schools, workplaces, and other community facilities)

Table 9-2 continues

Table 9-2 (*Continued*)

- Provide incentives to Food Stamp recipients to purchase more healthful and less energy-dense nutrient-poor foods and beverages
- Provide incentives for, or remove taxes on, the purchase of exercise equipment
- Formulate national campaigns to reduce television viewing
- Provide federal funding to state and local health departments for mass media health promotion campaigns
- Regulate advertising to increase health-promoting messages relative to those for energy-dense nutrient-poor foods and beverages

Education

- Educational materials regarding healthy weight management, based on research regarding content and delivery formats, must be developed for various age and socio-economic groups, and made more readily accessible. The focus of these materials should be on health rather than appearance, including the hazards of excess weight and weight gain, and the benefits of modest weight loss.

- Educate the public on the hazards of unhealthful methods of weight loss.

- Provide parental programs, aimed at helping children to increase their physical activity and to adopt healthy nutritional patterns, while enhancing positive attitudes within the family towards a healthy lifestyle and body weight.

- Health care providers, teachers, parents, and other community leaders should receive more education stressing the importance of achievable and healthy rather than unattainable and unrealistic weight loss, and guard against fad diets, disordered eating, and other unhealthy approaches to weight management.

- Physical education and health education must be increasingly incorporated into schools at all levels.

- Education programs should be developed to inform and motivate the population to adopt health-promoting practices.

- Official, focused training programs should be developed to create a field of obesity specialists whose profession deals exclusively with issues related to obesity treatment and prevention.

Prevention

- Greater attention must be focused on the prevention of obesity in all age groups to slow the rise in obesity prevalence and reduce associated health risks.

- Aspects of culture, including general lifestyles and attitudes that promote obesity should be challenged and reoriented toward more healthy patterns.

- National nutrition and physical activity policies should be developed that relate specifically to the prevention of obesity.

- Involvement and action from community organizations should increase to enhance positive societal attitudes and behaviors related to a healthful diet and physical activity.

Treatment

- Individualized multidisciplinary models should be developed, tested and implemented to maximize cost-effectiveness and practicality.

- Realistic health-related goals rather than cosmetic ideals must be established, beginning with modest weight losses (5–10%), which can result in significant risk factor reduction and improved health.

- Health care delivery systems that currently do not cover obesity treatment should carefully reassess this policy.

- Expenses incurred by treating comorbidities of obesity such as hypertension, coronary heart disease, dyslipidemias, type 2 diabetes and osteoarthritis should be considered in the economic decisions related to treating obesity.

Research

- Identify, develop, and test practical, efficacious, and cost-effective interventions and programs to prevent obesity.

- Identify economic and behavior patterns that will enable individuals and populations to adopt healthy diet and physical activity habits.

- Improve methodologies for monitoring diet, physical activity, and health-related behaviors and outcomes in various subpopulations, as well as methods to assess the effectiveness of interventions.

- Conduct randomized trials to address questions regarding the development of rational clinical and public health approaches to obesity.

CONCLUSIONS

As the obesity epidemic continues to gain momentum in most of the industrialized world, increased burdens are placed on health, economics, and quality of life. The ongoing escalation of overweight and obesity worldwide calls for major concerted efforts on the part of health care professionals from clinical, scientific, and public health standpoints, as well as governmental and community leaders. Because of the complex multifactorial etiology of obesity, solutions must be aimed at all the underlying factors, particularly unhealthy excessive dietary intake, physical inactivity, and sedentary lifestyles. Populations at increasing risk for obesity and its comorbidities, which may require particular focus, include groups with lower SES, racial ethnic minorities, children, adolescents, and the aging population. The Healthy People 2010 Goals provide specific targets that must be proactively and strategically worked towards during this decade. Policies promoting healthy weight must be implemented from federal, state, and local governments as well as the private sector, aimed at preventing further surges in the prevalence and severity of obesity. Population-based improvements in health-related attitudes and behaviors must be achieved, and environments must be geared toward promoting better daily diet and physical activity practices. Health outcomes, rather than aesthetic aspects of body weight, must be emphasized. Through education, prevention, treatment, and research, strides can be made to reverse one of the most serious health problems of our time.

REFERENCES

1. World Health Organization. Obesity: preventing and managing the global epidemic. Report of a WHO Consultation presented at: the World Health Organization; June 3–5, 1997; Geneva Switzerland. Publication WHO/NUT/NCD/98.1.
2. Dietary guidelines for Americans. Washington, DC: US Department of Health and Human Services, 1996.
3. Mokdad AH, Serdula MK, Dietz WH, Bowman BA, Marks JS, Koplan JP. The continuing epidemic of obesity in the United States. JAMA 2000; 284: 1650–1651.
4. National Institutes of Health. Clinical guidelines on the identification, evaluation, and treatment of overweight and obesity in adults: the evidence report. Bethesda, MD: National Heart, Lung and Blood Institute, June 1998.
5. Mokdad AH, Serdula MK, Dietz WH, Bowman BA, Marks JS, Koplan JP. The spread of the obesity epidemic in the United States, 1991–1998. JAMA 1999; 282: 1519–1522.
6. Must A, Spandano J, Coakley EH, Feild A, Colditz G, Dietz W. The disease burden associated with overweight and obesity. JAMA 1999; 282: 1523–1529.
7. National Task Force on the Prevention and Treatment of Obesity. Overweight, obesity and health risk. Arch Intern Med 2000; 160: 898–904.
8. Wolf AM, Colditz GA. Current estimates of the economic cost of obesity in the United States. Obes Res 1998; 6: 97–106.
9. Fine JT, Colditz GA, Coakley EH, Moseley G, Manson JE, Willett WC, Kawachi I. A prospective study of weight changes and health-related quality of life in women. JAMA 1999; 282: 2136–2142.
10. Ford ES, Moriarty DH, Zack MM, Mokdad AH, Chapman DP. Self-reported body mass index and health-related quality of

life: findings from the Behavioral Risk Factor Surveillance System. Obes Res 2001; 9: 21–31.

11. Dwyer J. Policy and healthy weight. Am J Clin Nutr 1996; 63: 415S–418S.

12. Swinburn B, Egger G, Raza F. Dissecting obesogenic environments: the development and application of a framework for identifying and prioritizing environmental interventions for obesity. Prev Med 1999; 29: 563–570.

13. Yanovski JA, Yanovski SZ. Recent advances in basic obesity research. JAMA 1999; 282: 1504–1506.

14. Harnack LJ, Jeffery RW, Boutelle KN. Temporal trends in energy intake in the United States: an ecologic perspective. Am J Clin Nutr 2000; 71: 1478–1484.

15. Lin B-H, Frazao E. Nutritonal quality of foods at and away from home. Food Rev 1997; 2: 33–40.

16. Lin B-H, Guthrie J, Frazao E. Away-from-home foods increasingly important to quality of American diet. Washington, DC: Economic Research Service/USDA and FDA/US DHHS, 1999.

17. Jeffrey RW, French SA. Epidemic obesity in the United States: are fast foods and television viewing contributing? Am J Public Health 1998; 88: 277–280.

18. McCrory MA, Fuss PJ, Hays NP, Vinken AG, Greenberg AS, Roberts SB. Overeating in America: association between restaurant food consumption and body fatness in healthy adult men and women ages 19–80. Obes Res 1999; 7: 564–571.

19. Calorie Control Council. Light foods and beverages soar to new levels of popularity. Calorie Control Commentary 1996; 18: 3.

20. Ernst ND, Obarzanek E, Clark MB, Briefel RR, Brown CD, Donato K. Cardiovascular health risks related to overweight. J Am Diet Assoc 1997; 97: S47–S51.

21. Hill JO, Melanson EL. Overview of the determinants of overweight and obesity: current evidence and research issues. Med Sci Sports Exerc 1999; 31: S515–S521.

22. National Restaurant Association. Healthy choices important to restaurant patrons, although behavior doesn't always mirror concerns. Washington, DC: National Restaurant Association, 1993.

23. Malouf NM, Colaguiri S. The effects of McDonalds, Kentucky Fried Chicken and Pizza Hut meals on recommended diets. Asia Pacific J Clin Nutr 1995; 4: 265–269.

24. Wansink B. Can package size accelerate usage volume? J Marketing 1996; 60: 1–14.

25. Mills S. Foodservice trends: healthy portions. Restaurants USA. Magazine of the National Restaurant Association. 1998; Apr: 39–46.

26. 44th annual: 100 leading national advertisers. Advertising Age 1999; 27: S1–S46.

27. Government and industry launch fruit and vegetable push; but NCI takes back seat. Nutrition Weekly 1992; 22: 1–2.

28. Briefel RR, McDowell MA, Alaimo K, et al. Total energy intake of the US population: third National Health and Nutrition Examination Survey, 1988–1991. Am J Clin Nutr 1995; 62: 1072S–1080S.

29. US Department of Agriculture. Data tables: results from USDA's 1994–96 continuing survey of food intakes by individuals and 1994–96 diet and health knowledge survey. December 1997. http://www.barc.usda.gov/bhnrc/food survey/home/htm

30. Frazao E. America's eating habits: changes and consequences. Washington, DC: US Department of Agriculture, 1999: Information Bulletin AIB-750.

31. Kant AK. Consumption of energy-dense, nutrient-poor foods by adult Americans: nutritional and health implications: third National Health and Nutrition Examination Survey, 1988–1994. Am J Clin Nutr 2000; 72: 929–936.

32. McCrory MA, Fuss PJ, Saltzman E, Roberts SB. Dietary determinants of energy intake and weight regulation in healthy adults. J Nutr 2000; 130: 276S–279S.

33. Gallo AE. First major drop in food product introductions in over 20 years. Food Rev 1997; 20: 33–35.

34. Nestle M, Jacobson MF. Halting the obesity epidemic: a public health policy approach. Public Health Rep 2000; 115: 13–24.

35. Bidlack WR. Interrelationships of food, nutrition, diet and health: the National Association of State Universities and Land Grant Colleges White Paper. J Am Coll Nutr 1996; 15: 422–433.

36. Koplan JP, Dietz WH. Caloric imbalance and public health policy. JAMA 1999; 282: 1579–1581.

37. US Department of Health and Human Services. Physical activity and health: a report of the Surgeon General. Atlanta: US Department of Health and Human Services, Centers for Disease Control and Prevention, National Center for Chronic Disease Prevention and Health Promotion, 1996.

38. Battle EK, Brownell KD. Confronting a rising tide of eating disorders and obesity: treatment vs. prevention and policy. Addict Behav 1996; 21: 755–765.

39. Foreyt J, Goodrick K. The ultimate triumph of obesity. Lancet 1995; 15: 134–135.

40. Wright JD. Triumph of obesity or of human insanity. Lancet 1995; 2: 637.

41. Fontanarosa PB. Patients, physicians, and weight control. JAMA 1999; 282: 1581–1582.

42. Serdula MK, Mokdad AH, Williamson DF, Galuska DA, Mendlein

JM, Heath GW. Prevalence of attempting weight loss and strategies for controlling weight. JAMA 1999; 282: 1353–1358.

43. Pasman WJ, Saris WHM, Westerterp-Plantenga MS. Predictors of weight maintenance. Obes Res 1999; 7: 43–50.

44. Winkleby MA, Fortmann SP, Barrett DC. Social class disparities in risk factors for disease: 8-year prevalence patterns by level of education. Prev Med 1990; 19: 1–12.

45. Martikainen PT, Marmot MG. Socioeconomic differences in weight gain and determinants and consequences of coronary risk factors. Am J Clin Nutr 1999; 69: 719–726.

46. Grembowski D, Patrick D, Diehr P, Durham M, Beresford S, Kay E, Hecht J. Self-efficacy and health behavior among older adults. J Health Soc Behav 1993; 34: 89–104.

47. Jeffery RW. Population perspectives on the prevention and treatment of obesity in minority populations. Am J Clin Nutr 1991; 53: 1621S–1624S.

48. Kumanyika SK. Obesity in minority populations: an epidemiological assessment. Obes Res 1994; 2: 66–184.

49. Kuczmarski RJ, Flegal KM, Campbell SM, Johnson CL. Increasing prevalence of overweight among US adults: the National Health and Nutrition Examination Surveys, 1960–1991. JAMA 1994; 272: 205–211.

50. Troiano RP, Flegal KM. Overweight children and adolescents: description, epidemiology, and demographics. Pediatrics 1998; 101: 497–504.

51. Johnson RK. Changing eating and physical activity patterns of US children. Proc Nutr Soc 2000; 59: 295–301.

52. Robinson TN. Reducing children's television viewing to prevent obesity. JAMA 1999; 282: 1561–1567.

53. Brady LM, Lindquist CH, Herd SL, Goran MI. Comparison of children's dietary intake patterns with US dietary guidelines. Br J Nutr 2000; 84: 361–367.

54. Troiano RP, Briefel RR, Carroll MD, Bialostosky K. Energy and fat intakes of children and adolescents in the United States: data from the National Health and Nutrition Examination Surveys. Am J Clin Nutr 2000; 72: 1343S–1353S.

55. Freedman DS, Dietz WH, Srinivasan SR, Berenson GS. The relation of overweight to cardiovascular risk factors among children and adolescents: the Bogalusa Heart Study. Pediatrics 1999; 103: 1175–1182.

56. Whitaker RC, Wright JA, Pepe MS, Seidel KD, Dietz WH. Predicting obesity in young adulthood from childhood and parental obesity. N Engl J Med 1997; 337: 869–873.

57. Must A, Jacques PF, Dallal GE, Bajema CJ, Dietz WH. Long-term morbidity and mortality of overweight adolescents: a follow-up of the Harvard Growth Study of 1922–1935. N Engl J Med 1992; 327: 1350–1355.

58. Gortmaker SL, Must A, Perrin JM, Sobol AM, Dietz WH.

Social and economic consequences of overweight in adolescence and young adulthood. N Engl J Med 1993; 329: 1008–1012.

59. Crandall CS, Schiffhauer KL. Anti-fat prejudice: beliefs, values, and American culture. Obes Res 1998; 6: 458–460.

60. US Bureau of the Census Current Population Reports, 1996. Washington, D.C.: US Bureau of Commerce.

61. Koplan JP, Fleming DW. Current and future public health challenges. JAMA 2000; 284: 1696–1698.

62. Lewis CE, Jacobs DR, McCreath H, Kiefe CI, Schreiner PJ, Smith DE, Williams OD. Weight gain continues in the 1990s: 10-year trends in weight and overweight from the CARDIA Study. Am J Epidemiol 2000; 151: 1172–1181.

63. Harris TB, Savage PJ, Tell GS, Haan M, Kumanyika S, Lynch JC. Carrying the burden of cardiovascular risk in old age: associations of weight and weight change with prevalent cardiovascular disease, risk factors, and health status in the Cardiovascular Health Study. Am J Clin Nutr 1997; 66: 837–844.

64. Guidance for treatment of adult obesity. Bethesda, MD: Shape Up America! and the American Obesity Association, 1996.

65. Carek PF, Sherer JT, Carson DS. Management of obesity: medical options. Am Fam Physician 1997; 55: 551–558.

66. Friedrich MJ. More healthy people in the 21st century? JAMA 2000; 283: 37–38.

67. Marwick C. Healthy people 2010 initiative launched. JAMA 2000; 283: 989–990.

68. Perusse L, Chagnon YC, Weisnagel SJ, Rankinen T, Snyder E, Sands J, Bouchard C. The human obesity gene map: the 2000 update. Obes Res 2001; 9: 135–169.

69. Weinsier RL. Genes and obesity: is there reason to change our behaviors? Ann Intern Med 1999; 130: 938–939.

70. Flegal KM, Troiano RP. Changes in the distribution of body mass index of adults and children in the US population. Int J Obes 2000; 24: 807–818.

71. French SA, Story M, Jeffery RW, Snyder P, Eisenberg M, Sidebottom A, Murray D. Pricing strategy to promote fruit and vegetable purchase in high school cafeterias. J Am Diet Assoc 1997; 97: 1008–1010.

72. French SA, Jeffery RW, Story M, Hannan P, Snyder M. A pricing strategy to promote low-fat snack choices through vending machines. Am J Public Health 1997; 87: 849–851.

Chapter 10

Obesity Research in the New Millennium

Risa J. Stein, C. Keith Haddock,
Walker S. Carlos Poston II,
and John P. Foreyt

The past 30 years of obesity research has been characterized by many changes in treatment design and delivery (1).
The number of treatments that have been tested for obesity
is impressive; researchers have been quite creative in their
attempt to discover a therapy that produces sustained weight
loss. However, if success in obesity treatment research is
defined as significant weight loss that is maintained indefinitely, our vast array of therapies have produced disappointing results. Foreyt (2) in reviewing the obesity literature
concluded that "obesity appears to be very difficult to treat
and there are no prospects of a long-term solution or cure
on the near horizon". Foreyt's comments suggest the need
for researchers to think in terms of different treatment
paradigms (3). In this chapter we outline several trends we
predict will characterize obesity research of the future. Some
of these trends have a long history while others require
changing our paradigms about obesity treatment.

CHANGING THE GOALS OF OBESITY TREATMENTS

Given that traditional obesity treatment programs do not produce sustained reductions in weight, researchers are reconsidering the reasons for using pounds lost as the benchmark criteria for success in obesity treatment as well as whether a different indicator of success may be more meaningful and achievable. Perhaps more important indicators of "success" in obesity treatment would include medical, psychological, and behavioral measures (4).

Historically, obesity researchers have justified their craft by pointing to the improvement in health parameters following weight loss rather than by the questionable goal of helping patients reach a subjective aesthetic standard. Therefore, it seems reasonable that weight loss would evolve to be, at best, a secondary outcome in obesity treatment research. As more obesity specialists advocate treatment programs that improve health-related indices rather than focus on body weight, sheer measurement of pounds lost (usually with the accompanied goal of reaching a societally influenced ideal weight) will continue to fall upon disrepute. Future research will attempt to develop treatments that are designed to improve health parameters rather than to promote weight loss *per se* (5).

PROMOTING BODY ACCEPTANCE

It will be difficult to socially market obesity programs focused on health rather than pounds lost if the primary reason patients pursue treatment is to improve their appearance. Therefore, future research should be directed toward developing treatments that reduce the level of weight obsession and the seemingly desperate attempt to control weight seen in many patients (5). There is a growing realization that body weight is not readily malleable, even on a short-term basis. For instance, a 1990 study by Stunkard et al (6) of 93 monozygotic twins reared apart found that 77% of the variance in body weight could be accounted for by genetics. Moreover, the amount of weight gain while on a fixed calorie diet and body fat distribution patterns are both influenced considerably by genetics (7). Thus, the control an obese individual can exert over their weight may be significantly limited. Patients who harbor unrealistic expectations eventually run up against their biological limits and inevitably suffer a blow to their self-esteem.

Given that most patients will not be able to reach and maintain their ideal body weight, a more relaxed and realistic approach to treatment which focuses on health seems reasonable, at least to professionals. However, a large body of evidence suggests that patients primarily join obesity treatment programs to improve their appearance through large weight losses. For instance, Foster et al (8) asked 60 obese women involved in a treatment program to define their goal weight losses. These women defined their goal weight loss as a 32% reduction in body weight, an objective quite different from the 5–10% reduction usually suggested by health professionals. These researchers also asked their patients about factors that influenced the selection of their goal weights. The principal reasons given for the selection of weight loss goals were appearance and physical comfort. Finally, although these women lost weight at a rate that would be considered quite reasonable in the obesity literature (i.e. 16 kg in 48 weeks), most patients reported dissatisfaction with their weight loss following treatment. Thus, developing successful obesity programs that encourage patients to focus on health rather than weight loss is likely to be a difficult, albeit important, undertaking.

FOCUS ON EXERCISE AND FITNESS

Physical exercise has been linked to a large number of medical and psychological benefits, including the promotion of healthy body composition (9). In terms of obesity, studies have demonstrated that exercise alone may be the preferred treatment for obesity (10,11). Regular exercise offers several important benefits for obese patients, including facilitation of energy release from adipose tissue (12), reduction of hypertension (9), reducing preference for dietary fats (13), and increased adherence to healthy eating habits (14). Furthermore, regular physical activity may mitigate many of the health concerns associated with obesity in those who remain overweight (15).

Additional research efforts are necessary to determine how best to involve the obese in physical activity and how to help them maintain exercise as a new habit. Obese patients who are working to develop a healthy exercise habit need to master several new skills (16). They need to become comfortable with sensations of perspiration, increased heart rate and breathing rate as well as the ability to change their schedules to accommodate exercise. Dunn et al (17) suggest that obese individuals who lack time and access to facilities and who profess a dislike of vigorous structured exercise may receive comparable benefits from moderate intensity lifestyle activity practised at least 30 min/day for most days of the week. Moreover, King et al (16) advocate providing ample social support at early stages of exercise incorporation because benefits are slight and discomfort is often high.

Exercise should be presented to patients as a method to promote health, energy, and fitness rather than weight loss. Patients should learn that moderate exercise that can be maintained, rather than extreme exercise goals, results in improved health and weight control as well as decreased attrition and injuries (18). Monitoring changes in health parameters (e.g. blood lipids, hypertension) and mood (e.g. depression) rather than body weight during an exercise program may provide incentives for overweight patients to continue physical activities despite slow or no changes in weight.

One very promising model for increasing exercise participation involves home-based programs (19–21). Home-based exercise programs are based on the presumption that exercising at home facilitates long-term adherence to exercise goals because the new skills are gained in and incorporated into the patient's natural environment. Added to the fact that most individuals prefer to exercise on their own rather than in a group format (20), home-based exercise programs provide an exciting line of obesity research. Perri et al (19) directly compared a traditional group exercise program with a home-based treatment in a group of obese women. At follow-up, patients in the home-based program demonstrated more exercise participation, greater treatment adherence, and significantly greater weight losses than those in the traditional group exercise program. Future obesity treatments should exploit the benefits of home-based programs and determine which specific factors are related to the success of these programs (e.g. supportive family environment, location, and time of exercise).

TREATMENT AS A LIFE-LONG PROCESS

"Cure" is perhaps an outdated notion iatrogenic to obesity treatment. Brownell (1) states that if "cure" is defined as weight loss to ideal body weight and maintenance of that weight status for 5 years, then "the cure rate for most forms of cancer is greater than that for obesity". Instead of the outdated notion of curing obesity with a specific time-limited treatment, new approaches will likely stress a "chronic" or "continuous care" model of obesity similar to that applied to the management of diabetes (18,22). Such a model would de-emphasize the promotion of long-term results based on a single treatment attempt and would instead espouse directing patients on how to rebound after episodes of overeating and gaining weight, thus continuing weight management across the lifespan.

Fairburn and Cooper (23) point out two significant barriers to the on-going maintenance of weight loss. First, many treatment programs do not teach weight maintenance behaviors or do not monitor the implementation of maintenance strategies. This barrier to weight maintenance could be overcome by replacing short-term treatments with a continuous care model similar to that used for diabetes or hypertension (22). In fact, we suggest that a continuous care plan implemented and rigorously monitored following initial treatment be adopted as a new standard of care for obesity treatment. Secondly, because most patients do not reach their ideal weight following treatment, many are unmotivated to maintain a weight loss they consider inconsequential. This barrier may be overcome with strategies designed to increase body shape acceptance. That is, if patients are able to enjoy the increased energy and fitness resulting from treatment and accept that they will not reach the cultural ideal of body shape, weight maintenance becomes more likely.

IDENTIFYING AND ADDRESSING PSYCHOSOCIAL PROBLEMS

Although a large body of research suggests that the obese do not have a higher prevalence of psychopathology compared to non-obese individuals (24,25), psychiatric comorbidities such as depression, low self-esteem, or eating disorders may moderate the effectiveness of obesity treatment. On the other hand, most behavioral weight loss treatment programs report improvement in psychological functioning during periods of weight loss (26). Binge eaters constitute one unique group of obese patients who have a relatively high prevalence of psychopathology (18). Future obesity treatment programs should screen for problems with binge eating because surveys have shown that 25–45% of individuals, depending on the criteria used, who present for obesity treatment report binge eating. Thus, the psychological presentation of the patient should play a part in the individualized development of obesity treatment strategies.

Both cognitive behavioral therapy (CBT) and interpersonal therapy (IPT) have demonstrated promise as effective treatments for psychiatric problems that may present comorbidly with obesity. CBT assumes that both styles of thinking and coping skills need to change in order to effect lasting changes in emotions and behaviors (27). IPT, while sharing several core features with CBT, suggests that negative effect and problematic behaviors are primarily the result of dissatisfaction with relationships and social impairment (28). Both of these therapies have demonstrated clinical and cost-effectiveness for psychiatric disorders such as depression, binge eating, and bulimic behaviors (29–31). Moreover, behavioral weight loss treatments have been demonstrated to decrease the frequency of binge eating episodes (26,32). Future obesity treatments will likely further integrate strategies to alter cognitive style and interpersonal functioning into current treatment modalities.

CONTINUED SEARCH FOR EFFECTIVE AND SAFE PHARMACOTHERAPIES

Drug therapies for obesity have long suffered from a negative public image and the withdrawal by the Food and Drug Administration (FDA) of two popular drugs, fenfluramine and dexfenfluramine, further tarnished the view of pharmacotherapies (33). In addition, recent FDA scrutiny of two pharmacological agents often found in appetite suppressants has further heightened public apprehension. A report that phenylpropanolamine, a stimulant, increased the probability of stroke in young women by more than 16 times has prompted FDA removal of the drug (34) and similar reviews currently threaten ephedra alkaloids (35). However, the development and prescription of drug treatments for obesity will likely continue. Several new pharmacotherapies are under study or have recently been granted FDA approval and will likely figure prominently in future treatment research. The new pharmacotherapies can be categorized as those which reduce energy intake, reduce nutrient absorption (nutrient partitioning), or increase energy expenditure.

Reduced Energy Intake

Sibutramine has been approved by the FDA while leptin and brain and gut peptides are under development as obesity therapies. Sibutramine, a norepinephrine and serotonin reuptake inhibitor has both satiating and thermogenic effects and produces weight losses of 4.7–7.6 kg in treatment trials lasting from 12 to 52 weeks (36). Leptin is a protein that may inhibit neuropeptide Y (NPY) gene expression and appears to increase satiety and energy expenditure. Leptin appears to control body weight through a feedback system which regulates fat storage. It has been. suggested that low levels of leptin may increase the risk for developing obesity. Unfortunately, several recent human studies demonstrated that obese individuals produce significant amounts of leptin, and that leptin levels are highly correlated with body weight (37,38). It is also possible that obese individuals are insensitive to endogenous leptin production, although there are currently no known defects in the leptin-effector system (38). It is also possible that premorbidly low levels of leptin predispose some individuals to develop obesity (39).

Brain and Gut Peptides Research has found elevated levels of β-endorphin in obese individuals when compared to lean subjects, findings that persist after weight loss (40). Elevated β-endorphin levels have also been found in binge eaters, regardless of their weight status (40,41). As a result, opiate peptide antagonists are now under investigation for applications to obesity and binge eating. For instance, naloxone, an opiate blocker, has shown promise in decreasing the desire for and consumption of sweet high-fat foods in binge eating women (42).

Nutrient Partitioning
Orlistat, a lipase inhibitor, produces significant (i.e. 4.74 ± 0.38 kg at a dosage of 360 mg/day after 12 weeks), dose-dependent weight losses (43–46). However, some patients report mild and transient gastrointestinal side-effects during treatment. Orlistat is approved by the FDA for the treatment of obesity.

Increased Energy Expenditure
β-3 agonists are under investigation for their ability to increase energy expenditure and produce weight loss. However, initial studies of the effectiveness of β-3 agonists for obesity have produced disappointing outcomes (47–49). β-3 agonists are currently not approved by the FDA for the treatment of obesity.

Although pharmacotherapies will continue to be an important clinical tool for the treatment of obesity, future research will need to address the poor adherence and attrition characteristic of these therapies. Attrition rates for clinical trials of obesity medications, even in specialty treatment centers, are substantial. If attrition is high in tightly controlled trials where considerable resources are often directed at reducing attrition and increasing compliance, it is likely to be a greater problem in other settings. Therefore, it is imperative that behavioral interventions specifically designed to increase compliance to obesity medications be developed. It may be that behavioral interventions designed to increase the patient's focus on health parameters, accept realistic weight loss, and increase acceptance of body shape would increase compliance with pharmacological interventions.

INCREASED RELIANCE ON PUBLIC HEALTH APPROACHES

Obesity is one of the most prominent public health problems in the United States. The prevalence of obesity has increased approximately 25% in the past 15 years (50). Currently, approximately 61% of U.S. adults are overweight or obese (51). The increase among ethnic minority groups has been even more dramatic, with 69% of African-American and 70% of Mexican-American women either overweight or obese (51). Given that over one quarter of the population is obese, it is unlikely that current treatments will reach the majority of overweight individuals. As a consequence, several researchers have suggested that future obesity research focus on public health approaches (52,53).

Public health approaches to obesity require the researcher to take a different perspective on the causes of obesity. Most current obesity treatments are based on the view that particular characteristics of individuals, such as genetics or a lack of control over eating, cause obesity. However, several factors strongly argue against the assumption that answers to the riddle of obesity are primarily found within the skin of our patients. The dramatic rise in the prevalence of obesity over the past decade cannot be explained by changes in the gene pool, with the presumption that successive generations have dramatically lower levels of self-control, or with the suggestion that people have recently learned to crave dietary fats and detest exercise. Also, treatments based on an individual approach have failed to stem the tide of obesity.

In contrast to the "within the skin" explanations of the rising tide of obesity, many researchers have argued that a paradigm shift is needed which looks to the environment for the causes of obesity (5,50,51). Many investigators have pointed to the "toxic environment" that has developed in industrialized countries as the principal reason for the high prevalence of obesity. For instance, Battle and Brownell (53, p. 761) suggest that "the environment provides access to and encourages consumption of a diet that is high in fat, high in calories, delicious, widely available, and low in cost" and that "with energy-saving devices and less physically demanding work, the number of individuals who maintain physical activity in day-to-day activities is diminishing".

How do we alter our "toxic environment" in order to increase the likelihood that the public will consume a healthy diet and remain physically active? Several regressive approaches have been suggested, such as controlling food advertising and increasing taxation on high-fat foods (5,52,53). However, it is questionable whether public support would exist for such efforts, because they may be viewed as infringements on one's right to determine one's own diet and activity level without intrusion by the federal government. For example, during congressional hearings (16 July 1997) Robert A. Levy of the Cato Institute stated:

> Proposals from supposedly intelligent people in positions of responsibility include grading goods for their fat content, taxing them accordingly, and using the revenues for public bike paths and exercise trails. When decisions about the products we choose to consume are entrusted to an unelected and unaccountable bureaucracy, the loss of personal freedom is inescapable. (54)

Public health interventions based on a non-regressive incentive-based approach may be more acceptable to the public (5,52,53). Healthy foods (i.e. fruits and vegetables) could be subsidized to encourage increased consumption, insurance companies could provide premium reductions on those who regularly exercise, and cities could receive grants to provide easily accessible and safe opportunities for physical activity (e.g. bike paths, well-maintained sidewalks, fitness centers). Also, private firms could be encouraged to provide fitness facilities and showers for their employees and allow workers to transfer sick leave to vacation time. Public health programs based on an incentive-based approach should receive increased attention in future obesity research.

CONCLUSIONS

The past three decades have seen great changes in treatments for obesity. However, despite extensive research in the area, few findings have significantly advanced the treatment of this condition. This chapter presents several courses of exploration which may redirect the area of obesity research toward novel and, it is to be hoped, more productive, avenues. Central to the current state-of-the-art treatment of obesity is a cognitive shift on behalf of providers as well as patients away from number of pounds lost and achievement of an aesthetic ideal to improved health and increased energy across the lifespan. Consistent with an emphasis on health, obesity researchers must continue to explore ways of involving the obese in regular, moderate, vigorous exercise programs. New areas of exploration will almost certainly involve pharmacological approaches to obesity management. However, public health approaches aimed at prevention and treatment of obesity through external agencies such as insurance premium reductions and exercise facilities provided by employers are likely to receive the most attention.

An integration of the new themes in obesity research suggests that an obese individual may experience the following when seeking treatment in the new millenium. First, he or she will be told that today's treatment programs take an individualized approach to care, which is likely to differ from the group programs he or she previously attended. This message will serve to emphasize that the practitioner is concerned about each individual and their health. Secondly, the chronic care approach will be outlined for the patient in a detailed fashion. Ideally, he or she will understand that weight management will be approached as a life-long process. Because treatment is framed as a continuous process across the lifespan, he or she will likely feel less stigmatized about returning for treatment following inevitable relapses and slips. As part of continued care, progress toward improved health, as well as the pros and cons of continued attempts at weight loss, will be routinely discussed with the health care providers.

One of the most prominent features of treatment will be the continual reinforcement of a cognitive shift toward self-esteem, independent of body weight. The program leaders will offer both social skills training and counseling on healthful methods of achieving nurturance and recognition. Instead of rapid weight loss goals achieved through severely restricted diet and acute strenuous exercise, a more gradual approach to increased health will be espoused. Gradual increases in exercise that are both pleasurable and vigorous will be coupled with a personally tailored diet that is modified in terms of composition but is not severely restrictive. After several weeks of treatment, the patient will most likely experience a 10% reduction in weight. However, during later treatment sessions the clinicians will primarily reinforce the decrease in blood pressure and the increase in physical fitness and energy the patient has experienced.

Once the initial treatment program is completed, the emphasis will be placed on maintenance of health and fitness gains. The patient will enroll in a comprehensive health maintenance program that is regularly monitored by area clinicians but is conducted at a local community center by volunteers. Periodically, he or she will return to the treatment program for medical check ups and "booster" sessions. Also, the patient's weight maintenance will be enhanced by a number of programs sponsored by local employers and the city government. For example, on warm days the patient will ride his or her bike to work on the newly constructed path through town. Fortunately, the employer installed a shower in the office area for individuals who either cycle to work or who exercise at lunch.

Maintaining the healthy diet the patient began during treatment is also easier because the company cafeteria instituted its healthy lunch program. High fat and calorie foods are hard to find at the cafeteria while inexpensive fruits and vegetables (subsidized by the company owner) are plentiful. Finally, a number of initiatives in his or her community and in the national media are sending the message that body weight and beauty are not necessarily linked. The patient is becoming convinced that, although not as skinny as the models that graced magazine covers during the 1980s and 1990s, he or she is attractive at his or her current weight. Healthy and fit models with a variety of body shapes grace the covers of popular magazines and television commercials.

Some may suggest that increasing patient acceptance of modest weight losses, incorporating public health approaches to weight management, and promoting positive changes in public attitudes toward varying body shapes could only occur in the fantasies of obesity researchers. However, in the course of three decades, cigarette smoking has evolved from a socially prized behavior that was sanctioned by sectors of the medical community to a deadly addiction which is viewed negatively by the public. The change in attitudes toward smoking was driven by dedicated public health and grass roots organizations that fought against prevailing public attitudes and an entrenched tobacco lobby. We are convinced that the obesity research community can accomplish similar goals.

REFERENCES

1. Brownell KD. Obesity: understanding and treating a serious, prevalent, and refractory disorder. J Consult Clin Psychol 1982; 50: 820–840.
2. Foreyt JP. Issues in the assessment and treatment of obesity. J Consult Clin Psychol 1987; 55: 677–684.
3. Beliard D, Kirschenbaum DS, Fitzgibbon ML. Evaluation of

an intensive weight control program using *a priori* criteria to determine outcome. Int J Obes 1992; 16: 505–517.

4. Atkinson RL. Proposed standards for judging the success of the treatment of obesity. Ann Intern Med 1993; 119: 677–680.

5. Foreyt JP, Poston WSC, Goodrick GK. Future directions in obesity and eating disorders. Addict Behav 1996; 21: 767–778.

6. Stunkard AJ, Harris JR, Pedersen NL, McClearn GE. The body-mass index of twins who have been reared apart. N Engl J Med 1990; 14: 249–258.

7. Bouchard C, Tremblay A, Despres JP, Naudeau A, Lupien PJ, Theriault G, Dussault J, Moorjani S, Pinault S, Fournier G. The response to long-term overfeeding in identical twins. N Engl J Med 1990; 322: 1477–1482.

8. Foster GD, Wadden TA, Vogt RA, Brewer G. What is reasonable weight loss? Patient's expectations and evaluations of obesity treatment outcomes. J Consult Clin Psychol 1997; 65: 79–85.

9. Pate RR, Pratt M, Blair SN, et al. Physical activity and public health: a recommendation from the Centers for Disease and Prevention and the American College of Sports Medicine. JAMA 1995; 273: 402–407.

10. Gwinup G. Effect of exercise alone on the weight of obese women. Arch Intern Med 1975; 135: 676–680.

11. Skender ML, Goodrick GK, del Junco DJ, Reeves RS, Darnell L, Gotto AM, Foreyt JP. Comparison of 2-year weight loss trends in behavioral treatment of obesity: diet, exercise, and combination interventions. J Am Diet Assoc 1996; 96: 342–346.

12. Bielenski R, Schutz Y, Jequier E. Energy expenditure and postprandial thermogenesis in obese women before and after weight loss. Am J Clin Nutr 1985; 42: 69–82.

13. Wood PD, Terry RB, Haskell WL. Metabolism of substrates: diet, lipoprotein metabolism and exercise. Fed Proc 1985; 44: 358–363.

14. Brownell KD. Exercise in the treatment of obesity. In: Brownell KD, Fairburn CG, eds. Eating disorders and obesity: a comprehensive handbook. New York: Guilford Press, 1995: 473–478.

15. Barlow CE, Kohl HW, Gibbons LW, Blair SN. Physical fitness, mortality, and obesity. Int J Obes Relat Metab Disord 1995; 19 (suppl 4): S41–S44.

16. King AC, Taylor CB, Haskell WL, DeBusk RF. Strategies for increasing early adherence to and long-term maintenance of home-based exercise training in healthy middle-aged men and women. Am J Cardiol 1988; 61: 628–632.

17. Dunn AL, Marcus BH, Kampert JB, Garcia ME, Kohl HW,

Blair SN. Comparison of lifestyle and structured interventions to increase physical activity and cardiorespiratory fitness: a randomized trial. JAMA 1999; 281: 327–334.

18. Foster GD, Kendall PC. The realistic treatment of obesity: changing the scales of success. Clin Psychol Rev 1994; 14: 701–736.

19. Perri MG, Martin D, Leermakers EA, Sears SF, Notelovitz M. Effects of group- vs. home-based exercise in the treatment of obesity. J Consult Clin Psychol 1997; 65: 278–285.

20. King AC, Haskell WL, Taylor CB, Kraemer HC, DeBusk RF. Group- vs. home-based exercise training in healthy older men and women. JAMA 1991; 266: 1535–1542.

21. King AC, Haskell WL, Young DR, et al. Long-term effects of varying intensities and formats of physical activity on participation rates, fitness, and lipoproteins in men and women aged 50–65 years. Circulation 1995; 91: 2596–2604.

22. Perri MG, Fuller PR. Success and failure in the treatment of obesity: where do we go from here? Med Exerc Nutr Health 1995; 4: 255–272.

23. Fairburn CG, Cooper Z. New perspectives on dietary and behavioural treatments for obesity. Int J Obes 1996; 20 (suppl 1), 9–13.

24. Friedman MA, Brownell KD. Psychological correlates of obesity: moving to the next research generation. Psychol Bull 1995; 117: 3–20.

25. Klesges RC, Haddock CK, Stein RJ, Klesges LM, Eck LH, Hanson CL. Relationship between psychosocial functioning and body fat in preschool children: a longitudinal investigation. J Consult Clin Psychol 1992; 60: 793–796.

26. National Task Force on the Prevention and Treatment of Obesity. Dieting and the development of eating disorders in overweight and obese adults. Arch Intern Med 2000; 160: 2581–2589.

27. Wessler RL. Conceptualizing cognitions in the cognitive-behavioral therapies. In: Dryden W, Golden WL, eds. Cognitive-behavioral approaches to psychotherapy. New York: Hemisphere Publishing, 1987: 1–30.

28. Agras WS. Non-pharmacological treatments of bulimia nervosa. J Clin Psychiatry 1991; 52 (suppl): 29–33.

29. Agras WS. Short-term psychological treatments for binge eating. In: Fairburn CG, Wilson GT, eds. Binge eating: nature, assessment, and treatment. New York: Guilford Press, 1993: 270–286.

30. Fairburn CG, Norman PA, Welch SL, O'Conner ME, Doll HA, Peveler RC. A prospective study of outcome in bulimia nervosa and the long-term effects of three psychological treatments. Arch Gen Psychology 1995; 52: 304–312.

31. Wilfley DE, Agras WS, Telch CF, Rossiter EM, Schneider JA,

Cole AG, Sifford L, Raeburn SD. Group cognitive behavioral therapy and group interpersonal psychotherapy for non-purging bulimics: a controlled comparison. J Consult Clin Psychol 1993; 61: 296–305.

32. Wilson GT. Cognitive behavioral therapy for eating disorders: progress and problems. Behav Res Ther 1999; 37 (suppl 1): 79–95.

33. US Food and Drug Adminstrations. FDA announces withdrawal of fenfluramine and dexfenfluramine. FDA Announcement, 15 September 1997.

34. Horwitz RI, Hines HH, Brass LM, Kernan WN, Viscoli CM. Phenylpropanolamine and risk of hemorrhagic stroke: final report of the hemorrhagic stroke project. 2000. http://www.fda.gov/cder/drug/infopage/ppa/default.htm

35. Haller CA, Benowitz NL. Adverse cardiovascular and central nervous system events associated with dietary supplements containing ephedra alkaloids. 2000. http://nejm.org/content/haller/1.asp.

36. Stock MJ. Sibutramine: a review of clinical efficacy. Int J Obes Relat Metab Disord 1997; 21 (suppl 1): 30–36.

37. Maffei M, Halaas J, Ravussin E, et al. Leptin levels in human and rodent: measurement of plasma leptin and ob RNA in obese and weight-related subjects. Nat Med 1995; 1: 1155–1161.

38. Considine RV, Sinha MK, Heiman ML, et al. Serum immunoreactive-leptin concentration in normal-weight and obese humans. N Engl J Med 1996; 334: 292–325.

39. Ravussin E, Pratley RE, Maffei M, et al. Relatively low plasma leptin concentrations precede weight gain in Pima Indians. Nat Med 1997; 3: 238–240.

40. Ericsson M, Poston WSC, Foreyt JP. Common biological pathways in eating disorders and obesity. Addict Behav 1996; 21: 733–743.

41. Drewnowski A. Metabolic determinants of binge eating. Addict Behav 1995; 20: 733–745.

42. Drewnowski A, Krahn DD, Demitrack MA, Nairn K, Gosnell BA. Naloxone, an opiate blocker, reduces the consumption of sweet high-fat foods in obese and lean female binge eaters. Am J Clin Nutr 1995; 61: 1206–1212.

43. Guerciolini R. Mode of action of orlistat. Int J Obes Relat Metab Disord 1997; 21 (suppl 3): 12–23.

44. Drent ML, van der Veen EA. Lipase inhibition: a novel concept in the treatment of obesity. Int J Obes Relat Metab Disord 1993; 17: 241–244.

45. Drent ML, Larsson I, William-Olsson T, et al. Orlistat (RO 18–0647), a lipase inhibitor, in the treatment of human obesity: a multiple dose study. Int J Obes Relat Metab Disord 1995; 19: 221–226.

46. Drent ML, van der Veen EA. First clinical studies with orlistat: a short review. Obes Res 1995; 3 (suppl 4): 623–625.

47. Connacher AA, Bennet WM, Jung RT. Clinical studies with β-adrenoreceptor agonist BRL 26830A. Am J Clin Nutr 1992; 55 (suppl 1): 258–261.

48. Connacher AA, Jung RT, Mitchell PE. Weight loss in obese subjects on a restricted diet given BRL 26830A, a new atypical β-adrenoreceptor agonist. Br Med J 1988; 296: 1217–1220.

49. Chapman BJ, Farquahar DL, Galloway SM, Simpson GK, Munro JF. The effects of a new beta-adrenoceptor agonist BRL 26830A in refractory obesity. Int J Obes Rel Metab Disord 1988; 12: 119–123.

50. Garfinkel PE. Forward. In: Brownell KD, Fairburn CG, eds. Eating disorders and obesity: a comprehensive handbook. New York: Guilford Press, 1995: vii–viii.

51. U.S. Department of Health and Human Services. The Surgeon General's call to action to prevent and decrease overweight and obesity. Rockville, MD: U.S. Department of Health and Human Services, Public Health Service, Office of the Surgeon General, 2001.

52. Jeffery RW. Public health approaches to the management of obesity. In: Brownell KD, Fairburn CG, eds. Eating disorders and obesity: a comprehensive handbook. New York: Guilford Press, 1995: 558–563.

53. Battle EK, Brownell KD. Confronting a rising tide of eating disorders and obesity: treatment vs. prevention and policy. Addict Behav 1996; 21: 755–765.

54. Levy RA. Global tobacco settlement. Statement of Robert A. Levy, PhD, JD, Senior Fellow in Constitutional Studies, Cato Institute, Washington, DC before the Committee on the Judiciary, United States Senate, July 16, 1997. Washington, DC: Cato Institute.

Index

Note: page numbers in *italics* refer to figures, those in **bold** refer to tables

A

abdomen
  adiposity 173
  fat deposition 3, 77
abdominal wall hernia 106
acanthosis nigricans 107
acarbose 118
acetosalicylic acid 119
activity factor (AF) 68, 69
adenosine triphosphatase (ATPase) 36
adiposity
  abdominal 173
  measures 194
  predictors 203
  see also fat, body; visceral adiposity
adolescents, obesity 231
adrenergic agonists 115–16, 128, 258
advertising, food 238
  budgets 226

control 260
aerobic exercise 37
  caloric intake impact 38–9
  weight maintenance 93
aerobic fitness 203
African Americans 230, 259
aging population 231–2
β-3 agonists 258
air displacement plethysmography 3
alcohol intake 75
Alström syndrome 205
American College of Sports Medicine (ACSM) 35
American Diabetes Association 180–1
American Heart Association (AHA)
  CHD risk factor 162
  healthy weight recommendations 77
American Obesity Association 80
amphetamines 107, **111**, 115
anemia, pernicious 66
anxiety 228
appearance-oriented goals 10, 253

appetite suppression 110
  exercise-induced 38, 39, 49
arthropathy 106, 107, 138
  see also osteoarthritis
aspirin 119, 128–9
assessment of obese patient 19–23
  ongoing 27–8
atherogenesis
  childhood obesity 196
  dyslipidemia 166–7
atherosclerosis, coronary 164
attitudes 230

B

back pain 149
basal metabolic rate (BMR) 67, 68
behavior, unhealthy 160–1
  see also sedentary behavior
behavior change strategies
  childhood obesity 206
  cognitive restructuring 89–91,
    95–7
  contingency management 88–9
  exercise 47
  family-based in childhood obesity
    206–7, **208–9**, 210–11
  integration in weight management
    plan 27
  medication compliance 259
  outcomes 211, **212–13**, 214
  refundable deposit contracts 89
  self-monitoring 47, 87–8, 94,
    98
  self-reward 88–9
  social support 91–2, 97
  stimulus control 86–7, 94, 98
  stress management 96–7
  weight loss 85–100
  weight maintenance strategies
    92–5
behavior disorders 21–2
behavior modification specialists 11,
    27
  integrated effort 15, *17*, 18
behavior therapy 99
beliefs 230, 235
  irrational 90
benzphetamine **111**, 115

biliopancreatic bypass, partial
    147–8, 149
binge eating 21
  cognitive behavioral therapy
    256–7
  disorder 79
  interpersonal therapies 256–7
  opiate peptide antagonists 258
bioelectrical impedance 8
Blackburn Model for Obesity 61,
    62
blood pressure
  reduction 13
  see also hypertension
body acceptance promotion 252–3,
    256
body composition 159
body mass, fat-free 37, 159
body mass index (BMI) 2–3, **4–7**, **8**
  childhood obesity 194
  cholesterol association 167
  combined therapies 59
  coronary heart disease association
    162
  diabetes type 2 association 168,
    169
  dyslipidemia association 162, 167
  gastric surgery eligibility 142
  increase 236
  lower socioeconomic status groups
    229
  measurement 18
  mortality association 159, *160*
  REE conversions 68–9
  stroke risk 163
  threshold for drug treatment 122
breast cancer 107, 138, 176, 177
bulimia nervosa 21, 116, 256

C

caffeine 114, 118, 119, 128–9
calcium
  deficiency 144–5
  dietary reference intakes 64–5
  loss in biliopancreatic diversion
    148, 149
  low calorie diet 75, **76**
  supplementation 77

calories/caloric intake
  counting 94
  decrease 34
  diets 60
  lifestyle activity 39–40
  low-calorie diet 75, **76**
  low-fat foods 74–5
  reduced availability 114
cancer 176–7
Cancer Prevention Study I 177, 180
carbohydrate intake 74–5
cardiac rehabilitation 49–50
cardiorespiratory fitness 50, 161
cardiovascular disease 66, 138, 149,
      156–82
  childhood obesity 196
  comorbidity 106
  dietary plan 79
  economic burden 232
  mortality 157, 162
  risk 161–4
  weight management in risk
      reduction 179–81
  see also coronary heart disease
      (CHD)
cardiovascular risk factors 157,
      164–76, 171
  childhood obesity 231
  clustering 170–1
  degree of weight loss 175–6
  hemostasis 170
  weight gain in middle age 232
Carpenter syndrome 205
catechin 119
catecholamines 108
Centers for Disease Control and
      Prevention 224
  healthy people goals 233–4
central nervous system abnormalities
      107
central obesity 172
  syndrome 140
cereals
  folic acid fortification 66
  see also grains
cervical cancer 176
childhood obesity 193–215, 231
  definition 194

etiology 198–205
implications 195–7
prevalence 193, 194–5
public policy 238
treatment 205–7, **208–9**, 210–11,
      212–13, 214
chitosan 114–15, 118
chlorphentermine 115
chlortermine 115
cholecalciferol 65
cholesterol/total cholesterol
  BMI association 167
  dietary control 167
  physical activity 49
  risk reduction with weight loss
      175–6
  weight regain 176
cirrhosis
  comorbidity 106
  J-I bypass 142
citrate lyase inhibition 115
clinical complications 232
coffee beans 119
cognitive behavioral therapy 256
cognitive distortion assessment 90–1
cognitive restructuring 89–91
  behavior change strategies 92–3
  strategies 95–7
cognitively-based procedures 48–9
Cohen syndrome 205
colon cancer 107, 138, 176
communication in multidisciplinary
      team 18, 25, 27
comorbid conditions 21, **22**, 23,
      106–7
  childhood obesity 231
  economic burden 244–5
  gastrointestinal disturbance 106
  improvement with drug treatment
      123
  prevalence **158**
  resolution with gastric surgery
      149–50
  severe 151
  see also cardiovascular disease;
      diabetes, type 2;
      dyslipidemia; hypertension;
      osteoarthritis; sleep apnea

computed tomography (CT) 3
confusion 228–9
congestive heart failure 163–4
contingency management 88–9
contracts, refundable deposit 89
coronary heart disease (CHD) 11,
        138, 149
    BMI association 162
    childhood obesity 195, 214
    economic burden 244
    risk 171
        factors 85, 162
        reduction 179–81
    weight
        gain 174
        management 179–81
cost–benefits of exercise 45, 46–7
counseling 12
cultural factors 240
cultural practices 230
Cushing's syndrome 205
cytomel 121

D

decision balance sheets 45–7
depression
    childhood obesity 197
    cognitive behavioral therapy 256
    interpersonal therapy 256
    monitoring 254
    social support 91–2
dexfenfluramine 107, 110, 114,
        128
    withdrawal 257
diabetes, type 2 11, 138, 140, 149
    BMI correlation 162, 168, 169
    childhood obesity 195
    comorbidity 106
    dietary plan 79
    economic burden 232, 245
    gastric surgery 148
    liver condition association 178
    risk factors 168–70, 171
    visceral adiposity correlation 168
    weight loss effect 169–70, 175,
        181
    weight regain risk 169
diaries, activity 26

diet
    attitude adjustment 10
    behavioral adjustment 10
    change promotion 71–2, *73*, 74,
        94
    childhood obesity 205–6, 207,
        208–9, 210
    classifications 59–61
    composition 25, 74–5, **76**, 77
    energy content 25
    fad 78–9
    healthful 237, 244, 260–1
    hypocaloric 207, **208**
    improper 12
    integration in weight management
        plan 27
    lifestyle management 61, *62*
    low calorie 60, 61, *62,* 64
        calcium intake 65
        step I 75, **76**, 77
    monitoring chart 72, *73*, 74
    nutrition adequacy 63–7
    nutritional considerations 25–6
    physical activity 61, *62*
    protein-sparing modified 207
    public policy 235
    qualitative improvement 63, 235
    suitability 25
    traffic light 207, **209**, 210
    very low calorie 60–1, *62*
    weight loss 74
    see also eating; food; nutrition
dietary choice 40
    improvement 239
dietary factors in mortality 227
dietary folate equivalent (DFE) 66
dietary habits, unhealthy 226–7
dietary-induced thermogenesis (DIT)
        114
dietary intake
    assessment 22
    estimation 71–2, *73*, 74
dietary management 58–81
dietary overconsumption 9
dietary reference intake
    calcium 64–5
    folic acid 65–7
    vitamin B_{12} 67

dietary supplements 77, 118
dietary treatment model 61, *62*, 63
  seven-step process 80–1
diethylpropion **111**, 116
dieting, yo-yo 21
dietitians 11
  diet monitoring 61, *62*
  integrated effort 15, *16*, 18
digestive enzyme inhibition 114
Digi-Walker digital step counter 71,
  74
discouragement 228–9
disease, chronic 11–12
disease risk, chronic **8**
drug treatment 106–30
  categories of drugs 115–21
  combination 128–9
  compliance 125
  criteria for receiving 121–2
  dosage **111–13**, 124, 125
  energy intake reduction 110,
    111–13, 114
  mechanisms of action 110,
    111–13, 114–15
  non-responders 125–6
  research 257–9
  responders 125–6
  results 126–9
  side effects 124
  single drug trials 126–8
  starting doses **111–13**, 124
  supportive 23
dual energy X-ray absorptiometry
  (DEXA) 3
dumping syndrome 144
duodenal switch operations 148–9
dyslipidemia 166–8
  BMI as risk factor 162, 167
  childhood obesity 195
  coronary heart disease risk 171
  economic burden 244–5
  weight loss 175, 180

E

eating
  automatic responses 87
  lack of control 259
  meal patterns 77–8
  patterns 75
  portion size 226
  positive behaviors 87
  rate slowing 93
  restaurant food 226
  triggers 86
  see also diet; food; nutrition
eating disorders 21–2
  see also bulimia nervosa
economic burden 232–3
education
  public policy 235, 237, 243–4
  see also health education; patient
    education
education level, lower 229–30
emotions, negative 228
employers **241–2**, 261, 263
employment 107
  sick days lost 232
endocrinopathies 107
  childhood obesity 205
endometrial cancer 176, 177
β-endorphins 258
endothelial dysfunction 196
energy
  imbalance 203
  promotion with exercise 254, 256
  release from body fat 253
energy balance 25, 78, 235
  diet composition 75
  negative 109
  positive 228, 238
energy expenditure 34, 35–8
  balancing 235
  childhood obesity 199
  high-intensity exercise 211
  increase 10, 114, 258–9
  physical activity 35–6
  resting 36–8, 67, 68–9
  total (TEE) 67, 68
energy intake
  balancing 235
  daily 226–7
  etiology 198–9
  exercise-induced suppression 38
  moderation 10
  physical activity 39–40
  reduction 110, **111–13**, 114

energy intake (*cont.*)
  restriction 14
  underreporting 198
enteroglucagon 144
environmental factors 260
environmental opportunities 230
ephedra alkaloids 257
ephedrine 114, 118–19, 128–9
epidemic of obesity 224–5, 236–8
  reversing causes 234–5
exercise
  behavior change strategies 47
  childhood obesity 200–5, 205–6,
    208–9, 210–11
  children's levels 202
  cognitively-based procedures
    48–9
  convenience 95
  cost–benefits 45, 46–7
  energy consumption 39–40
  feedback 43–4
  focus 253–5
  frequency of intense bouts 37
  goal setting 42–3, 47
  health benefits 49–50, 254
  high-intensity 37, 38, 40, 210,
    211
  home-based 95, 254–5
  initiation improvement strategies
    41–4
  intensity 35–6, 37, **208–9**,
    210–11
    moderate 38, 40–1
  interval training 36
  maintenance
    difficulties 47–9
    strategies 41–4
  management 34–51
  physical benefits 49–50
  programs 22
  prompting 41–2, 48
  psychological benefits 49–50
  public policy 235, 237–8
  reinforcer withdrawal 48
  resting energy expenditure 36–8
  schools 227, 238, 243
  self-control procedures 48–9
  self-monitoring 47

visceral adiposity effect 214
  weight maintenance 93, 94–5
  see also aerobic exercise; physical
    activity
exercise physiologists 11
  integrated effort 15, *17,* 18

F

famine 108
fat, body
  central 20
  childhood obesity 194
  distribution 2–3, 253
  energy release 253
  mass 159
  patterning in children 196–7
  percentage 3, 8
  peripheral 18–20
  stores 75
  see also adiposity; visceral
    adiposity
fat, dietary 13
  absorption inhibition 118
  childhood obesity 199
  gram counting 94
  intake 74–5
    restriction 94
  monounsaturated 75
  oxidation 204
  preference reduction 253
  sedentary behavior association
    199
  substitutes 77
Federal Trade Commission (US)
  119
feedback, performance 43–4
feeding response 108
fenfluramine 107, 114
  phentermine combination
    116–17, 128
  withdrawal 257
fiber consumption 13
  low calorie diet 75, **76**
fibrinogen 170
fibrinolysis, impaired 170
fitness
  aerobic 203
  cardiovascular 211

focus 253–5
gain 262
physical 13
promotion with exercise 254
weight maintenance 256
flour, folic acid fortification 66
fluoxetine 116, 117
  clinical trials 126–7
  phentermine combination 128
folic acid
  dietary reference intake 65–7
  supplementation 65, 66, 77
food
  advertising budgets 226
  availability of healthy types
    239
  checklists 25–6
  childhood obesity 231
  classification 96
  craving 90
  daily record 72
  energy-dense nutrient-poor 227,
    231, 237
  healthful 237, 244, 260–1
  healthy choices 87
  intake 75
    limitation 94
    self-monitoring 87–8
  labeling 237
  meal patterns 77–8
  overconsumption 9
  portion sizes 72, 77–8, 87
  problem 96
  quantity limitation 94
  records 25–6
  restaurant 226, 237
  snack 238
  spending 226
  subsidies 261, 263
  taxation 260
  thermic effect 67, 68, 199, 200
  vendors 237
  see also diet; eating; nutrition
Food and Drug Administration (US)
    119, 122
  antiobesity drug withdrawal 257
  drug approval 123
  food labeling 237

Food Guide Pyramid 63–4, 66
  portion sizes 72
food industry 236–7
  health food 119
Framingham Heart Study 162, 163
  diabetes protection 169
  risk factor clustering 170–1
fruit consumption 13, 65, 66,
    260–1
  availability of affordable types
    239
  children 231
  encouragement 237
functional capacity 13

G

gall bladder disease 106, 138, 178
  cancer 107, 176
gallstone formation 145, 178
Garcinia cambogia 115, 120
gastrectomy, subtotal 147
gastric banding procedures 146–7,
    149
gastric bypass (GBP) 142, *143*,
    144–7, 149
  laparoscopic 147
gastric surgery 142, *143*, 144–7
gastroesophageal reflux 140, 146,
    149
gastrointestinal absorption, drug-
    induced decrease 114–15
gastrointestinal disturbance
    comorbidity 106
gastroplasty, horizontal 146–7
gastroplasty, vertical banded (VBGP)
    142, *143*, 144–7
genetic disorders, childhood obesity
    205
genetic factors 259
  body fat distribution 253
  predisposition to obesity 225,
    234–5
  weight variance 252
genitourinary cancers 107
glucose
  fasting blood levels 13
  fasting serum 21
  gastric surgery 144

glucose intolerance
  BMI correlation 168
  childhood obesity 231
  visceral adiposity correlation 168
glucose tolerance
  impaired 169
  risk reduction with weight loss
    175
goal setting 10, 18, 23
  distal 42–3
  exercise 42–3, 47
  fixed 42, 43
  flexible 42, 43
  proximal 42–3
  self-monitoring 44, 47
  self-setting 43
government recommendations
  242–3
grains
  folic acid fortification 66
  whole 239
green tea extract 119
growth, energy costs 198
growth hormone (GH) deficiency
  107

H

health
  benefits of physical activity 49–50
  maintenance 262
  monitoring of parameters 254
  outcomes 2, 9–10, 240
  promotion 254
  public policy 235
  risk 3, 21, **22**
health care
  costs 232–3
  delivery systems 244
  providers 243
  services **241**
health education 235, 237
  access 230
  public policy 243–4
health food industry 119
Health Maintenance Organizations
  (HMOs) 150–1
Health Professionals Follow-up
  Study 162

health status 21
  improvement 27–8
healthy people goals 233–4
heart rate monitor feedback 43–4
height 2, **4–7**
  measurement 18
hemostasis, cardiovascular risk 170
hernia incidence 106, 140
  gastric surgery 147
hiatus hernia 106
high density lipoprotein (HDL) 166,
  167
  childhood obesity 195, 197
  dietary control 167, 168
  risk reduction with weight loss
    175
  visceral adiposity 172, *173*
  weight regain 176
Hispanic Americans 230
hunger
  exercise-induced suppression 38,
    39, 49
  reduction 110
hydrodensitometry 3
hydroxycitric acid 115, 120
hyperadrenalism 107
hypercholesterolemia 149, 231
hyperfibrinogenemia 107
hyperglycemia 140, 168
hyperhomocystinemia 66
hyperinsulinemia 107, 120, 164
  BMI correlation 168, 169
  childhood obesity 195
  coronary heart disease risk 171
  liver condition association 178
  visceral adiposity 168, 169
hypertension 11, 138, 140, 149
  BMI as risk factor 162
  cardiovascular risk factor 164–6
  childhood obesity 195
  comorbidity 106
  coronary heart disease risk 171
  dietary plan 79
  economic burden 232, 244
  monitoring 254
  obesity association 165–6
  physical activity 49
  reduction with exercise 253

weight gain association 165
weight loss 175, 180
  effectiveness 164–5, 166
weight regain 176
hypogonadism 107
hypothyroidism 107, 205
hypoventilation 138, 140, 149, 178

I

insulin
  childhood obesity 197
  gastric surgery 144
  hypersecretion 169
  resistance 120, 164
  risk reduction with weight loss
    175
  sensitivity 120
  see also hyperinsulinemia
insulin resistance 172
  BMI correlation 168, 169
  visceral adiposity 168, 169, 172
interpersonal therapy 256
intertrigo 107
interval training 36
intestinal bypass 142
intra-abdominal pressure, increased
    140, 150
intracranial pressure, increased 140
Iowa Women's Health Study 172
iron deficiency 144–5

J

jejunoileal (J-I) bypass 142
Joint National Committee (JNC) VI
    Guidelines 180
joint pain 149

L

Laurence–Moon–Biedl syndrome
    205
left ventricular dysfunction 163–4
  childhood obesity 196
leisure time 227
leptin 121, 204–5, 257–8
life expectancy 239
lifestyle
  activity 39–40, 49–50, 95
  change 11, 25

eating habits 210
factors 225–6
healthy 210, 230
management 11, 23, **24**, 25–7
  diet 61, *62*
modification 98–9
mortality association 12
permanent changes 2
promotion of healthier 235
sedentary 9, 12, 227–8
therapy 59
unhealthy behaviors 160–1
weight management 18–23, **24**,
    25–8, 79–80
linoleic acid, conjugated 119
lipase inhibition 258
lipid blood levels
  diet therapy 167
  fasting 13
  monitoring 254
lipids
  oxidation 204
  plasma 170
  profile 21
lipogenesis 115, 120
liver conditions 178–9
liver function tests 21
longevity 108
low density lipoprotein (LDL) 166,
    167
  childhood obesity 195, 197
  dietary control 167–8
  risk reduction with weight loss
    175–6
  small dense particles 166–7, 172
lung disease, obstructive 107

M

Ma Huang 119
magnesium 120
magnetic resonance imaging (MRI)
    197
maladaptive behaviors 89–90
mass media 235
mazindol **113**, 116
  clinical trials 126, **127**
meal patterns 77–8
meal replacements 77

Medicaid 150–1
medical professionals **241**
medication *see* drug treatment
Metabolic Measurement Cart
    Horizons Systems 68
metabolic profile 13
metabolic rate *see* basal metabolic
    rate (BMR); resting
    metabolic rate (RMR)
metamphetamines 115
metformin 120
methamphetamine **111**
metronidazole therapy 142
Mexicans 230, 259
Mifflin–St Jeor equation (MSJE)
    68
milk, non-fat (skim) 67
mobility in older age 232
mood state
    lifestyle activity 49
    monitoring 254
    see also depression
morbidity 138, **139**, 140
    work-related 107
    see also psychosocial morbidity
mortality
    all-cause 157, 159–61, 162
    BMI level 159, *160*
    dietary factors 227
    fat loss 160
multidisciplinary approach 1–2,
    13–15, *16–17*, 18
    integrated effort 15, 18
    lifestyle weight management
        18–23, **24**, 25–8
multidisciplinary team
    communication 18, 25, 27
    member roles 15
    physician role 25
    record keeping 18
    support follow-up 26, 28
multivitamin tablets 77
muscle mass increase 37

N

naloxone 258
National Cholesterol Education
    Program 167–8, 180

National Health and Nutrition
    Evaluation Survey
    (NHANES) III 156–7, 167,
    259
    childhood obesity 195, 199
    daily energy intake 226–7
    gall bladder disease 178
    osteoarthritis 177
    risk factor clustering 170–1
    television viewing 203
National Heart, Lung and Blood
    Institute (NHLBI) guidelines
    122, 123, 173
National Institutes of Health (NIH)
    3
    classification criteria for obesity
        156
    criteria for receiving drug
        treatment 121–2
    guidelines for treatment strategy
        selection 23, **24**
    treatment algorithm 14, 19, **20**
National Weight Control Registry
    93–4, 181
necrotizing panniculitis 138
networking, online 18
neural tube defects 65
neuropeptide Y (NPY) 108
    gene expression inhibition 257
night eating syndrome 21
norepinephrine 37
norepinephrine reuptake inhibitor
    257
North American Association for the
    Study of Obesity (NAASO)
    122
Nurses' Health Study 161, 162,
    177
nutrient partitioning 115, 258
nutrition
    barriers to improvement 22
    childhood obesity 206
    public policy 235, 244
    see also diet; eating; food
nutritional information provision
    237
nutritionists, diet monitoring 61,
    62

O

obesity
  BMI **4–7**
  classification 3, **8**
  definition 3
  etiology 9
  management 239
  medical condition 11–13
  prevalence 224, 225, 259
  prevention 236–8, 239, 244
  severity 225
  specialty field 244
  status 8–9
opiate peptide antagonists 258
orlistat **113**, 118, 258
  clinical trials 127–8
osteoarthritis 21, 107, 138, 177
  economic burden 232, 245
osteoporosis 148
ovarian cancer 176
over-weight
  BMI **4–7, 8**
  classification **8**
  definition 3
oxygen, maximal consumption 203

P

parenting styles 206
patient
  communication with
    multidisciplinary team 25
  follow-up 27–8
  individual needs 25
  integrated effort 15, *16,* 18
  lifestyle change integration 25
  readiness to change 21, 22
  regular visits 27–8
  self-monitoring 18, 26, 47
  self-motivation 22
  support follow-up 26
  unrealistic expectations 253
  weight management behavior
    improvement 25, **26**
patient compliance 11, 88
  decision balance sheet use 46
  drug treatment 125
  exercise convenience 95

exercise intensity 211
  medications 259
patient education 129
  resources 26, 80, 243
pedometers 71, 74
peripheral obesity syndrome 140
pernicious anemia 66
personal factors 240
phendimetrazine **111**, 115
phentermine **112–13**, 116
  fenfluramine combination
    116–17, 128
  fluoxetine combination 128
phenylpropanolamine (PPA) 107,
    116, 257
phosphate 120
physical activity 10, 34–5
  activity factor 69
  barriers to 22
  childhood obesity 200–6, **208–9,**
    210–11
  combined therapies 59
  diet 61, *62*
  diminishing 260
  efficiency of body 36
  effort intensity **70**
  energy
    balance 67, 68
    consumption 39–40
    expenditure 35–6, 199
  feedback 43–4
  focus 253–5
  goal setting 42–3
  health benefits 49–50
  improved 13
  increased 14
  initiation
    difficulties 40–1
    improvement strategies 41–4
  integration in weight management
    plan 27
  intensity 203
    moderate 38, 40–1
  maintenance
    difficulties 40–1, 47–9
    strategies 41–4
  medical evaluation 26
  monitoring 69, 71, 74

physical activity (*cont.*)
  prompting 41–2, 48
  public policy 235, 237–8, 244
  reinforcer withdrawal 48
  schools 227, 238, 243
  weight maintenance 94–5
  see also exercise
physical fitness, improved 13
physical inactivity 226, 227–8
physicians 9, 11, 12
  dietary treatment 61
  integrated effort 15, *16*, 18
  obesity treatment 13
  screening candidates for drug
      treatment 122
  weight management 13
    multidisciplinary programs 15,
      25
  weight reduction advice 12
Pickwickian syndrome 107, 138
  gastric surgery 148
Pima Indians 204
pituitary dysfunction 107
plasminogen activator inhibitor 1
    (PAI-1) 170
plethysmography, air displacement
    3
polycystic ovary syndrome 107
portion size 226
potassium 120
Prader–Willi syndrome 205
pregnancy complications 107
primary care 9, 61
  see also physicians
problem-solving techniques 45–50
PROCAM study 167
program adherence 46
prompting 41–2
  self-monitoring of diet 88
  withdrawal 48
prostate cancer 138, 176
protein, dietary
  high biological value 60
  lean sources 239
  low calorie diet 75, **76**
  vitamin B_{12} intake 67
protein–calorie malnutrition 148,
    149

pseudohypoparathyroidism 205
pseudotumor cerebri 138, 140, 149
psychosocial morbidity 107, 140
  childhood obesity 197
  problem identification 256–7
public health 224–6
  incentive-based approach 261
  messages 235
  potential models 238–40
  recommendations 240, **241–3**
  research 259–61
  special populations 229–32
public policy 235, 236–8
pulmonary embolism 138

Q

quality of life 13, 151
  multidisciplinary approaches
      13–14

R

racial ethnic minorities 230, 259
recidivism 9, 92
  avoidance 11, 181
  food classification 96
  incidence 140, 142
  prevention 9, 28
record keeping, multidisciplinary
      team 18
recreation 227
relapse *see* recidivism
renal disease 107
research in obesity control 245,
    251–63
  body acceptance 252–3
  drug treatment 257–9
  physical activity 253–5
  psychosocial problems 256–7
  public health 259–61
  treatment
    goals 252
    life-long process 255–6
respiratory failure 107
resting energy expenditure (REE)
    36–8, 67, 68–9
resting metabolic rate (RMR) 114
  childhood obesity 199–205
risk–benefit analysis 99

Roux-en-Y operation *see* gastric
bypass (GBP)

S

schools
  health education 243
  physical activities 227, 238, 243
sedentary behavior 227–8
  dietary fat intake 199
  lifestyle 9, 12, 227–8
  public policy 235
selective serotonin reuptake
      inhibitors (SSRIs) 116, 117,
      257
self-control procedures 98–9
  exercise 48–9
self-efficacy 13, 40, 230
self-esteem 13, 197
  cognitive shift 262
self-help treatment 63
self-instructional training (SIT) 90
self-monitoring 18, 26
  behavior change strategies 47,
      92–3, 94, 98
  behavioral strategies 87–8
  diet 72, *73*, 74
  exercise 47
  prompts 88
  weight loss 88
self-perception 197
self-reinforcement in behavior
      change 92–3
self-reward 88–9
self-worth 197
serotonin agonists 110, 116, 128
serotonin syndrome 117
sertraline 116
sex hormone imbalance 140
sibutramine **113**, 117, 257
  clinical trials 127
sick days lost 232
skin infections 138
skinfold measurement 3, 8
  childhood obesity 194
sleep apnea 21, 107, 138, 149,
      177–8
smoking 159
social factors 240

social influence program 93
social practices 230, 235
social support 91–2
social trends 235
societal attitudes 244
socioeconomic status, lower 229–30
sodium
  insulin-induced resorption 140
  renal retention 164
soft drinks 231, 237
soft-tissue infections 107
spending on food 226
spouse participation 91
steatohepatitis, non-alcoholic 179
stigmatization 240, 262
stimulus control 86–7
  behavior change strategies 92–3,
      94, 98
stress 228
  management 96–7
stress incontinence 138, 140
stroke, BMI association 163
subsidies for foods 261, 263
success evaluation 99
sugar substitutes 77
sunlight 65
surgery/surgical interventions 59,
      138–51
  complications 107
Swedish Obesity Study (SOS) 151,
      165, *166*
sweet eaters 144, *145*
syndrome X 140, 172
  childhood obesity 195–6
  visceral adiposity 196, 197
  see also insulin resistance

T

tachyphylaxis 119, 124
taxation 260
telephone prompts 41
television watching 202–3, 231, 238
thermic effect of food (TEF) 67, 68,
      199, 200
thermogenesis 119, 120
  dietary-induced (DIT) 114
  peripheral 119
thermoregulation 198

thought processes 90
thyroid dysfunction 21
thyroid hormones 21, 108, 121
thyroid-stimulating hormone (TSH)
    21
thyroxine (T_4) 121
topiramate 120–1
total energy expenditure (TEE) 67,
    68
toxic environment 260
treatment
    access to services 230
    decisions 100
    effectiveness 99
    goals 10, 18, 23, 252
    individualized 2
    life-long process 255–6, 262
    NIH guidelines for strategy
        selection 23, **24**
    outcomes 13
    program integration 25
    public policy 244–5
    risk–benefit analysis 99
    see also drug treatment; patient
        compliance
Trials of Hypertension Prevention
    (TOHP I and II) 164–5
triglycerides 166, 167
    childhood obesity 195, 197
    dietary control 167
    risk reduction with weight loss
        175
    visceral adiposity 172, *173*
    weight regain 176
triiodothyronine (T_3) 108, 121

U

underweight, BMI **4–7**
urge overflow incontinence 138, 140
urinary bladder pressure 140, *141,
    150*
urinary incontinence 138, 140, 150
ursodiol 145
uterine cancers 138

V

values 235
varicose veins 107

vegetable consumption 13, 65, 66,
    260–1
    availability of affordable types
        239
    children 231
    encouragement 237
venous stasis ulcers 107, 138, 140,
    149
visceral adiposity 3, 163, 168,
    171–4
    coronary heart disease risk
        171–2, 196
    diabetes type 2 196
    exercise effect 214
    high density lipoprotein 172, *173*
    hyperinsulinemia 169
    insulin resistance 169, 172
    syndrome X association 196, 197
    triglycerides 172, *173*
    weight reduction 173–4
    see also fat, body
vitamin(s)
    deficiencies with gastric surgery
        148, 149
    supplementation 77, 118
vitamin B_{12}
    deficiency 66, 67, 144–5
    dietary reference intake 67
    supplementation 77
vitamin C supplements 77
vitamin D 65

W

waist circumference 3, 197
    classification **8**
    measurement 18
waist : hip ratio (WHR) 172, 197
walking 49–50
weight
    activity energy expenditure
        adjustment 201
    all-cause mortality association
        157
    BMI 2–3, **4–7**
    cycling 21
    healthy **4–7**
    measurement 18
    obsession 252

personal sensitiveness 240
variance 252
weight control 9–10
  evidence-based techniques 10
  strategies 93–4
weight gain
  avoidance in already obese 236
  breast cancer 177
  coronary heart disease 174
  genetic predisposition 75
  hypertension association 165
  mortality increase 161
  precipitants 21
  prevention 61, 63
  primary prevention 10
weight loss
  attempts 12
  behavioral strategies 85–100
  diabetes type 2 169–70, 175, 181
  diet 74
  dyslipidemia 175, 180
  education 243
  gastric surgery 145–6, 149
  goals 10, 129, 175, 243, 244
  group self-monitoring 88
  health risk factor amelioration 123
  hemostatic risk factors 170
  hypertension 180
    control effectiveness 164–5, 166, 175
  incremental 80
  intentional 161
  interventions 8–9
  lifestyle activity 49, 50
  maintenance 10, 14, 255–6
  mechanisms guarding against 108
  mortality decrease 161
  multidisciplinary approaches 13–14
  outcome 99
  parental involvement 211, 214
  protocol 23
  self-monitoring 88
  self-reward 88–9
  sleep apnea 178
  social support 91–2, 97

success criteria 122–4
timescale 14
visceral adiposity 174
weight maintenance 263–4
  aerobic exercise 93
  barriers 255–6
  cardiovascular risk 175–6
  exercise 93, 94–5
  failure 123
  groups 92–3
  lifestyle activity 95
  long-term 28, 59
  multidisciplinary approaches 13–14
  physical activity 94–5
  post-treatment contact 93
  social influence program 93
  social support 91–2, 97
  strategy 14, 92–5
  stress management 96–7
weight management 1, 9–11
  behavior improvement 25, **26**
  comprehensive program 129–30
  coronary heart disease risk reduction 179–81
  drug role 109–10
  lifestyle 18–23, **24**, 25–8
    approach 79–80
  misinformation 228–9
  multidisciplinary programs 12, 14–15
  physicians 13
  strategies 23
    integration 27
  treatment goals 18
weight regain 61, 108, 109
  antiobesity drug withdrawal 110
  blood pressure increase 176
  cholesterol levels 176
  diabetes risk 169
  high density lipoprotein 176
  prevention 63, 129
  sleep apnea 178
  triglycerides 176
work efficiency 36
work-related morbidity 107
World Health Organization (WHO) 3, 156, 173